Medicine and Business

Ronald V. Bucci

Medicine and Business

A Practitioner's Guide

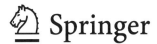 Springer

Ronald V. Bucci, PhD, MBA
Administration
Akron Children's Hospital
Akron, OH, USA

ISBN 978-3-319-04059-2   ISBN 978-3-319-04060-8 (eBook)
DOI 10.1007/978-3-319-04060-8
Springer Cham Heidelberg New York Dordrecht London

Library of Congress Control Number: 2014931368

Printed on acid-free paper

Springer is part of Springer Science+Business Media (www.springer.com)

Preface

The purpose of this book is to provide a baseline knowledge set of business admin-istration skills for physicians and individuals entering administrative positions in the healthcare field. More physicians are becoming leaders within the healthcare system and a growing number of physicians lead organizations. However, many of the physicians and nonphysicians entering administrative positions in hospitals and health systems lack the basic business administration skills that are required to per-form their duties in these positions.

Physicians do not normally acquire business administration skills during their medical training, and non-physicians may or may not receive business training dur-ing their academic instruction. Even if healthcare professionals have acquired advanced degrees in business administration, healthcare administration, nursing administration, or other professional programs, they may lack many of the business skills needed to operate a hospital or medical practice. Many of the abilities that are lacking include, but are not limited to, financial, organizational, and leadership exper-tise; understanding of the revenue cycle; and the knowledge and implications of healthcare policies, laws, and regulations that control the healthcare environment.

In developing this book, I have drawn on my work experience in different health-care settings, including hospitals and outpatient care facilities, private and public healthcare systems, and for-profit and not-for-profit businesses. Healthcare admin-istrators need training in business administration skills to properly and effectively perform their functions while providing "value" to their organization. While this book is not an in-depth educational tool for achieving proficiency in accounting, finance, or organizational management, it does provide a basic set of business skills that can be used in both the private and public healthcare sectors. It is tailored expressly for physicians and other healthcare professionals who are assuming administrative roles in these settings.

Medicine and Business: A Practitioner's Guide begins with an introduction to the relationships between business and healthcare and discusses the importance of lead-ership, mission creation, and governance to the success of healthcare organizations. Chapters 4–7 explain the purpose and interpretation of financial and income statements, balance sheets, and cash flows and detail the similarities and differences in these tools in healthcare and non-healthcare sectors. Financial analysis, budgeting, and business and strategic planning are described in Chapters 8–10, followed by a discussion about the types of health insurance, managed care, and payment methods (Chapters 11–15). Chapters 14 and 15 review business and hospital organizations and physician's compensation structures. The book concludes with an overview of medical business law and regulations and new government initiatives, such as the Affordable Care Act. Features of the book include instructional details about and illustrations of the development and analysis of financial statements as well as situational life examples derived from healthcare businesses.

The healthcare system and the roles of administrators in this system have changed dramatically over time. Historically, these positions did not require administrators to possess advanced business skills to be successful in their jobs. However, factors such as cost controls, managed care, and government regulations and oversight have permanently changed the healthcare system in the United States. These professionals need to be proficient in applying business administration and management strategies to their practice so as to insure the success, viability, and sustainability of their organizations.

In preparation for the actual development of this book, an advisory committee consisting of physicians, healthcare professionals, and a finance specialist was assembled. These individuals gave suggestions for content and reviewed portions of the writing to validate that it fulfilled the intentions of the author. This advisory committee included Michael Rubin, M.D.; Joseph Iemma, M.D.; Ibrahim Farid, M.D.; Russell Maroni; and Shana Locktish. I am grateful for these contributions to the book and also appreciate the support of my family, including my wife Lynn; my children Gina, Dominic, Angelo, and Maria; and our family dog Amber.

Akron, OH, USA   Ronald V. Bucci, PhD, MBA

Contents

Chapter 1
Healthcare and Business

Abstract Business and healthcare are two terms we hear almost every day, but rarely do we hear them together. Healthcare is the prevention, maintenance, or restoration of a person's health by trained medical specialists and medical institutions. Business is when a type of person or corporation of some sort sells goods or services in an effort to make a profit. Business and healthcare should be used together since one cannot survive without the other. A healthcare service must be treated like a business and make a profit so that it can pay its employees and vendors, while sustaining growth for an economically viable life. Healthcare has changed over time from a business where there is an excess of cash available to a business with increased regulation and governance, increased costs, and reduced cash flow. Managed care, the Joint Commission on Accreditation of Healthcare Organizations (JCAHO), state and federal regulations, the Centers for Medicare and Medicaid Services (CMS), the Patient Protection and Affordable Care Act (PPACA) or (ACA), the Health Insurance Portability and Accountability Act (HIPAA) of 1996, the Health Information Technology for Economic and Clinical Health (HITECH), accountable care, and many other factors make the healthcare business one of complexity and confusion. Our complex healthcare world demands that physician and nonphysician leaders develop an understanding of the business aspect of healthcare. These changes in healthcare have also caused alterations in healthcare leadership positions. Many physicians have been called upon to be leaders of healthcare organizations, and this trend is likely to continue as more and more physicians are becoming employees of healthcare systems. Many of today's leaders are experts at either the healthcare field or business, but not always both. This can be financially detrimental to a healthcare business. The chapters in this book are intended to assist in the education of healthcare leaders, including both physicians and nonphysician administrators, in the tools of the healthcare business trade. These tools will apply to both the for-profit side and not-for-profit side of healthcare. Not-for-profit businesses still need to make a "profit."

The US Healthcare Delivery System

Healthcare in the United States is an open market system that is unlike other health systems across the globe. Many other countries in the world have some type of national health insurance which is organized, controlled, and financed by the government. In most of those countries, the citizens are entitled to some type of health insurance. This is not the case in the United States. An actual controlled and regulated "system" does not exist. We have a fragmented or chaotic system with many different interests, pieces, and parts. People obtain healthcare and payments for healthcare through different means and avenues. Not everyone in the country is able to obtain health insurance or has access to healthcare services. Furthermore, patients do not always have a choice of physician or medical facility.

Part of the complexity of our system is the vast number of institutions and healthcare providers. The United States has a multitude of providers involved in the delivery of healthcare for primary, acute, auxiliary, extended, and continuing care. According to the US Census Bureau, there are 5,795 hospitals in the country and 38,453 active doctors of medicine, 70,480 osteopathic physicians, 12,900 podiatrists, 52,600 chiropractors, 86,000 dentists, and 2.5 million nurses (U.S. Census Bureau 2013). Many of these providers of healthcare work independently of each other.

Access and Financing

A highly developed healthcare system's four main goals should be:

- To enable citizens to have healthcare when needed
- To be of high quality
- To be cost-effective
- To have a mechanism for payment of services

Two parts of healthcare business are access and financing. Access refers to how services are delivered to patients by providers. Access is very important to people in need of medical care. People may not have access to healthcare providers due to not having insurance, inability to get to a provider, wait times to get into a provider, or a number of other reasons. The other part of healthcare is financing. Financing is how patient care is paid for. It can be paid by a multitude of resources including government, private insurance, and patient cash out of pocket. How this access or lack of access works along with multiple payment options is what makes our healthcare system very complicated, inefficient, and ineffective. The administrator's job is to manage all of these resources and providers in order to take care of patients' needs and wants while at the same time maintaining enough of an income to keep the provider in business.

US Healthcare System Characteristics

The US health system does not operate in a rational and integrated way. It is more of a chaotic relationship between payers, financers, insurers, and delivery systems. There is also a blend of private and government providers and payers that make it even more complicated. Some of these include:

- A large array of healthcare settings where medical care services can be delivered
- An unstructured payment collection system among providers and insurers
- A vast number of insurance agencies, managed care organizations (MCO), and other types of insurers
- Multiple payers making up their own rules for insurance and pricing of services
- Too many consulting firms offering expertise and healthcare services

This fragmented and uncontrolled healthcare system has some unique challenges as well. Some of these are:

- Duplication and overlap of services
- Provider inefficiencies and a waste of resources among providers
- Inconsistencies and inadequate healthcare services
- The largest healthcare system in the world (too large to be controlled by a single force)
- Inadequate controls of patient care quality

The US healthcare system has some unique characteristics that make the system good in some instances of healthcare but very complicated and confusing to manage. These different characteristics include governance of the system, third-party payers, technology, and patient care quality.

No Governing Bureau

The US healthcare system is not controlled or operated by any department or agency of the government. Most other countries have a central control of healthcare services. The system is financed both by the public and by government organizations, and there are a variety of payments, insurances, and delivery systems. This lack of control causes chaos in the healthcare business. The services provided, the price charged, and the choice of who to provide services for are all fair and open grounds for the provider to do as they choose. The provider can choose what to provide, when and where to provide it, and how much to charge for it. The government programs such as Medicare and Medicaid do have rules and regulations, but providers still have the choice of whether or not to be contracted with these programs.

Unbalanced Access of Care

"Access to care or healthcare services" is the ability for an individual to obtain healthcare services when needed. In the United States, this access is limited to people who have:

- Health insurance provided by their employer
- Health insurance provided by government services
- Health services paid by the consumer or the consumer's personal resources
- Health services obtained from free clinics and other free providers

The services available to an individual are determined by which of these categories that individual belongs. Each of these situations predetermines where a patient can get services, when a patient can get services, what services are available, and how much the patient will have to pay out of their own pocket. The product of such a system is a society where access and quality of care is unbalanced between different groups.

Unfree Market

A free market can exist in many businesses. Some of the characteristics of a free market are that the buyers and sellers act independently; people are able to pick and choose who they work with and buy from; the patients would be able to make free choices of doctors and hospitals; prices for services would be negotiated between the buyer and the seller; prices for services would be known to both the patient and provider; free competition would exist; and the patients would have a free choice of service set. This is not the case in the US healthcare system. The buyers and sellers or providers of health services and healthcare do not work independently of each other. A third party such as a government-sponsored healthcare plan or private insurance plan usually works in between the patient and provider and makes decisions such as the patients' provider and the price of services. This takes the freedom of choice away from the patient and provider regarding who can have services and when those services will be provided. In regard to the price setting, historically, Medicare and Medicaid have taken the initiative to set prices for healthcare services. The rest of the market normally follows this pricing pattern in some manner. Competition among providers seems to be dwindling because of two effects. The first effect is that conglomerates among healthcare organizations are being formed and thus have taken over regions of the market. The second force is the trend of physicians being employed by healthcare systems. This trend removes the physician as a competitor to a healthcare system and instead makes them part of it. Also, in our healthcare market, prices for services are not normally available for the consumer to examine. This can be envisioned by the patients as unforeseen or hidden costs. One example would be that a patient will be billed for the professional interpretation of the x-ray exam along with the cost to take the x-ray itself. While this billing structure is predetermined by the insurer, this may appear to be a duplicate charge to the patient. Finally, in this market, the patient does not always directly bear the responsibility of the payment of the procedure since it is normally borne by a third-party or government payer.

Payers

In countries where there is a national healthcare system, the government exists as the single payer for the entire system. In the United States, we have multiple payers available to our citizens. These can be third-party insurance companies, managed care organizations, and government payers such as Medicare and Medicaid. This multi-payer system has its disadvantages. Some of these are:

- It can be almost impossible for a consumer to keep up on all health plans available to them along with what the benefits are for each of these plans. There are just too many plans to keep track of.
- The billing practices of providers are not standardized. Each payer, including third-party payers and the government, institutes their own standards, policies, and procedures for authorization of services and then the billing and payment of the services. A provider of services must be able to work with all these different payers and their unique systems.
- Payers of services have a unique process of denying claims for variety of reasons along with specific plans on how to appeal and re-bill for these denials.
- Providers of services have many challenges when collecting certain bills for patients. The collection process is lengthy and costly since it can involve issuing time collection letters and then turning the accounts over to a collections agent.
- Our government programs which include Medicare and Medicaid have very complex rules and regulations and generally stretch out the time from billing to payment over a longer period of time than other payers.

Legal Risks

The United States can be described as overutilizing the legal system in regard to lawsuits against people. The medical system is part of this challenge in that there have been a large number of lawsuits filed for services rendered by doctors and hospitals. This has caused our medical system to practice defensive medicine, over utilizing diagnostic information and over supplying patients with cures for their conditions. Many of these additional efforts may not be necessary, which can raise the cost and inefficiency of the healthcare system.

Technology and Quality

Many feel that our healthcare system has the highest-quality patient care in the world, as well as the best technology and equipment, to take care of our patients. Research and innovation in medical technology is more prominent in the United States than in the rest of world. This is both a positive and a negative for the health-care system. The positive side is that our system does produce high-quality patient care which can be seen by the increase in our average life span. Our citizens are able to live healthier and more productive lives in our current generation of healthcare than in the past. Along with this benefit of our system come the cost of all this tech-nology and quality and the burden of a larger population with a higher age demo-graphic, which requires more and more medical care.

Significance of Healthcare Business Management

While we seem to have the best healthcare system in the world in regard to taking care of our citizens and technology and quality, our system is quite complex, redun-dant, inefficient, and costly to our country. The healthcare manager of today, whether it is a physician or a nonphysician, needs to work with all these characteristics of the US healthcare system to produce a high-quality work in a cost-effective manner while making a profit for their organization.

An administrator in the healthcare arena needs to have a good understanding of the US healthcare system and its ramifications so they can make critical decisions in regard to operations, planning, and management. This is true for whether the com-pany is a for-profit or a not-for-profit company. The areas of significance that need to be accounted for are as follows:

Healthcare delivery—The system of healthcare providers, from private physician offices to large hospital networks, needs to be understood in its entirety, from how these companies are organized and operated to the operational incentives for these institutions.

Financial well-being—Today's healthcare administrator needs to be able to look at their company and determine its financial health and viability both as a company alone and in comparison to other companies in the industry.

Financing—The administrator should be able to understand two sides of financing. The first side is how payments are billed and received for services rendered. The second side is how to apply these payments as well as other forms of income such as grants, subsidies, and investments into the maintenance, research, growth, and expansion of the facilities' services.

Strategic planning—The organization needs to review itself using the SWOT analy-sis approach, which consists of an analysis of the company's strengths, weaknesses, opportunities, and threats. This will be described in a later chapter of this book. This information is key in developing a plan for growth and overall sustainability of your healthcare business. Business and strategic planning are essential in any viable company.

Organizational positioning—Whether your organization is a small single physician practice or a large organization, it fits into the overall macro market of healthcare in some respect. The administrator should realize where in the environment they fit, as well as where the organization wishes to be in the future. Along with this, you should also be aware of how the outside environment, including legislative, competition, and overall healthcare environmental actions and developments will affect you and your organization now and in the future.

Healthcare policy—Within the healthcare administrator, there should be an understanding of how the healthcare policy system works in this country, at both the federal and state levels. Policy decisions at both of these levels affect how the organization is operated, regulated, and paid for services. Healthcare leaders need to stay current on laws that are passed and laws that are pending and be proactive on new laws that should be addressed in the future.

Regulations—Healthcare is regulated at the federal and state level by government departments such as the Centers for Medicare and Medicaid Services or your state Department of Health, as well as by organizations that we are members of, such as the American Medical Association or the American Hospital Association. Regulations affect every aspect of how we conduct business in our healthcare institutions. Compliance with these legal and voluntary institutions is vital to the continued operation of any healthcare business. Noncompliance can deter your level of operations, cut programs, cut access to valuable sources, and even force closure of your business.

Administrators in the healthcare business are vital to the long-term success of that business. The better administrators will have an understanding of both healthcare and business. These two words cannot act independently or the business will be a failure. A firm that can provide high-quality medical service but is unable to bill and collect revenue for services will not be a financial success; and a firm that has the billing and revenue collection mastered but is unable to provide good medical care for its patients also will be a failure. A combination of both aspects working together has the best chance of success in this business. Administrators in healthcare will be both physicians and nonphysicians. Whichever one it is, they will need to acquire the knowledge and skills of business to be successful administrators.

Further Reading

Barton P. Understanding the U.S. health services system. Chicago, IL: Health Administration Press; 2010.

Buchbinder S, Shanks N. Introduction to health care management. Burlington, MA: Jones & Bartlett Learning; 2012.

Census.gov. US Census Bureau. (Online) http://www.census.gov/. Accessed 8 Oct 2013.

Fallon L, Mcconnell C. Human resources management in health care. Burlington, MA: Jones & Bartlett Learning; 2014

Griffith J, White K. The well-managed healthcare organization. Chicago, IL: AUPHA Press; 2002.

Mcconnell C, Umiker W. Umiker's management skills for the new health care supervisor. Burlington, MA: Jones & Bartlett Learning; 2014.

Niles N. Basics of the U.S. health care system. Sudbury, MA: Jones and Bartlett; 2011.

Rubino L, Esparza S, Chassiakos Y. New leadership for today's health care professionals. Burlington, MA: Jones & Bartlett Learning; 2014.

Shi L, Singh D. Delivering health care in America. Sudbury, MA: Jones & Bartlett Learning; 2012.

Shi L, Singh D. Essentials of the U.S. health care system. Burlington, MA: Jones & Bartlett Learning; 2013.

Sultz H, Young K. Health care USA. Burlington, MA: Jones & Bartlett Learning; 2014.

Chapter 2
Leadership and Governance

Abstract Healthcare organizations such as medical practices, clinics, and hospitals operate with a set of principles or foundation blocks. These principles are normally part of the vision and mission statements of a company. The mission and vision chart the course of action in day-to-day operations and future business planning and development. Leadership is then called upon to implement these principles and guide your organization to be successful in its mission. Strong leadership in any business setting is critical to the success of that organization. These leaders will perform their functions in different leadership styles, but all leaders need to learn how to be good. Some may argue that some leaders are born and some leaders are created. In reality, this is a mixture of both, but in any case, all good leaders need to learn the fundamentals of leadership and then continually educate themselves and learn from experiences to be a better leader in the future. John F. Kennedy once said, "Leadership and learning are indispensable to each other." Governance is how the leadership and the company are organized. There are different types of governance structure, depending on the size and type of organization. Hospital systems will have a board of directors as their governance, while a small medical practice may just have the physician as the president of the company and a less structured governance system. The governance team, the mission and vision of the hospital, and the leadership team must all be in sync together to be a successful organization.

Leadership Versus Management

Leadership is the ability to create an environment based on guidance, respect, and empowerment of the people to act consistently in the direction of the mission of the organization. Leadership deals more with influencing, motivating, and enabling others to be successful in the organization. Leaders have followers. Leaders are more of the charismatic or transformational style where they coach, mentor, and enable their people for success.

R.V. Bucci, *Medicine and Business: A Practitioner's Guide*, 9
DOI 10.1007/978-3-319-04060-8_2, © Springer International Publishing Switzerland 2014

Table 2.1 Leadership role types in healthcare

Organization type	Sample positions
Physician practice	Physician president
	Practice manager
	Office coordinator
	Billing supervisor
Clinic or outpatient center	Chief administrative officer
	Human resources manager
	Director of admissions
	Supervisor of housekeeping
Hospital or healthcare system	President/CEO
	Chief medical officer
	Chief nursing officer
	Vice president
	Director of pharmacy
	Supervisor of maintenance

Management is the coordination and oversight of the business division or task in order to accomplish desired goals and outcomes of an organization. Management deals with directing and controlling individuals or groups to accomplish goals. They focus more on goals, structure, and human resources. Managers have subordinates. Managers use more of an authoritative or transactional style, where they tell the people what to do and how to do it.

The definitions of leadership and management are very similar yet are also very different. They are both driving individuals to desired results, but their approach to the accomplishment is different. If you are in an administrator's position, are you a leader or manager or both? The difference between managers and leaders is philosophical. It can be said that managers manage processes and leaders lead people. In other words, a manager is a person who achieves their desired results by working through people in more of a bureaucratic approach. Leaders work with their employees and coworkers by encouraging communication and feedback to accomplish their goals. This text will focus on the leadership model that is needed in healthcare.

Leadership

Leaders can play many roles in the organization. They are put in positions of authority in the organization to lead the people to carry out the mission. They not only ensure that patients receive adequate and high-quality care, they must assure that this care is appropriate, timely, and effective, while meeting the financial goals and mission of their organization. There are many different kinds of roles in management. They can vary from company to company, from industry to industry, and are also dependent on the size and the corporate structure as well. Some different roles and leadership are displayed in Table 2.1.

Physician Leadership

Over time, there has been a transformation in the leadership of healthcare systems from nonphysician leaders to physician leaders. Traditionally, in smaller operations such as medical clinics and physician offices, the physician has always been the top-ranking administrator in their office, and they had a very limited formal management structure. In a larger, hospital-type atmosphere, administrators have mainly been people with healthcare and/or business-type backgrounds. The typical hospital administrator would have been someone with a healthcare background that pursued educational goals of a Master of Business Administration or a Master of Nursing and then moved up the ranks. Over time, there has been an increase in physicians becoming administrators in hospitals and other types of healthcare businesses. Examples of this include physician CEO's of major institutions such as the Cleveland Clinic, Duke Medical System, or UCLA Health System. Physicians are filling positions such as the CEO, COO, vice president's, and department leaders in hospitals. This trend has increased in proportion to the movement of physician employment from independent physician to employed physicians.

Physician Leadership Skills

Physicians go through many years of school, residency, and internships before they are able to practice medicine. During all this training, the focus is in medical training in order to care for a patient in their discipline. There has never been a traditional focus on training in skills needed for business and hospital administration. Physicians may depend on outside consultants such as accountants, attorneys, and business managers who they hire to operate their practices. This philosophy has changed over time to where the physician needs to learn and use business administration skills in any type of practice or employment that they enter into. Physicians can now be tasked with the financial analysis of the business, the understanding and use of contracts, managed care, and growing a business if they are in administrative positions.

Non-physician Leadership Skills

Many current administrators of hospitals, medical practices, and clinics have been either people who have started out as nurses or some type of technician and have moved up through the ranks of the company into management positions or individuals who have focused their education on Masters Programs of Health and Hospital Administration and have moved straight into an administrative role. While many of these people seem to be educated in healthcare and/or business, additional skills and training are needed for them to be successful in today's world of healthcare. A nurse or a respiratory technician who moves up to an administrative level may not know how to look at an income statement or balance sheet in order to give a financial assessment of the company. They may not know how to formulate a business plan in order to grow the business. These skills are normally learned through additional schooling, on-the-job training, or self-growth.

Leadership: Functions, Traits, Skills, and Actions

Leadership can mean many things to many people. Good leaders are individuals who believe in themselves and others as well. Leaders tend to create environments where people can use their talents and strengths to promote a productive working environment. A good leadership environment is one where there is cooperation among individuals, groups, and organizations.

Functions

Some leadership functions are as follows:

Planning—This is a function of any management style. It requires the leader to review the mission, vision and goals of the company and form a strategic plan of how to achieve those goals. It is accomplished by setting priorities, targets, and a timeline.

Organizing—This function involves coordinating and orchestrating all resources of the organization, including people, plants, property, and equipment. It also involves the determination of positions, teams, relationships, and scopes of responsibility.

Decision-making—This is a critical function that seems basic but can be difficult for many people. People must be able to make wise decisions in order not to impede operations of the company. They will need to make decisions based on facts, vision, and observations in a timely manner.

Control—The leader must monitor the operations of the business and keep them in line with budgetary and strategic initiatives. The leader must realign the workforce in organizations when strategic alignment is out of place. A good leader also holds his people accountable for their actions and the results of their job.

Traits

Leaders are said to have good traits or bad traits in regard to managing and leading people. The following are a list of what can be considered good traits and another list of not-so-good or bad traits:

Good and bad leadership traits

Good traits	Bad traits
Inspirational	Incompetent
Ambitious	Rigid
Loyal	Insensitive
Transparent	Callous
Committed	Corrupt
Decisive	Temperamental
Energetic	Overreactive
Selfless	Rude
Humble	Lazy
Proud	Indecisive
Enthusiastic	Selfish
Humorous	Forceful
Consciousness	Offensive
Self-assured	Intimidating
Dominant	Overbearing

Skills

The following are skills that are necessary for a good leader. Many of these skills can be taught and acquired by leaders through training, education, and experience:

Communication	Business administration
Listening	Negotiation
Motivation	Conceptual
Interpersonal	Persuading
Coaching, mentoring, and training	Evaluation
Team building	Counseling
Relationship building	Leading by example
Development	Organization
Planning	Delegation
Decision-making	

Do's and Don'ts

Actions speak louder than words and your employees recognize this. The following is a list of some good actions and some bad actions presented by leaders:

Do's:

Always treat others as you want to be treated yourself.
Be loyal to your team and your organization.

Research and think before you make a decision.
Be respectful above and below you, as well as outside of you.
Lead with honor and respect.
Do the right action as opposed to the easy wrong one.
Lead by example.
Build relationships in both your area and outside areas.
Keep an open line of communication.
Always be transparent.
Empower your people.
Remember that democracy always rules.

Don'ts:

Don't be disrespectful.
Don't be overreactive.
Don't make decisions out of haste.
Don't speak in language that is unbecoming, unprofessional, and uncharacteristic
    of a leader.
Don't forget where you came from.
Don't fear in making decisions.
Don't intimidate or put fear in your people.
Don't humiliate people.
Don't push your blame on others.

Everyone has been asked at some point what type of leadership style they have
or what type of leader they are. There are different leadership styles, from autocratic
to participatory to coaching. Table 2.2 displays some of the more popular leadership
styles and definitions.

Leadership Styles

Governance

Governance can be defined as the system in which the organization or corporation
is directed and controlled. It defines who is in charge of the organization, the mission and vision, and delineates the organizational structure including the levels of
authority and responsibility. The size and scope of the governance body vary by the
type and size of an organization. Generally the size of most boards will be between
6 and 12 people and is composed of members from within and outside of the organization. A small physician's office probably will not have a board of directors, but
as corporations grow in size and complexity, there becomes a need to establish some
type of board for control of the organization. For-profit organizations will have a
board of directors that are made up of owners of the corporation and sometimes

Table 2.2 Leadership styles

Leadership style	Definition
Autocratic	A style in which the leader makes all decisions without any input from his staff. They possess total authority and use their power to force their substituents to complete their tasks. This style is most effective when the employees have close supervision
Laissez-faire	The laissez-faire type of leadership is one in which the leader gives very little feedback to the employees. It works well where the employees do not need much supervision and require very little input from the actual leader
Participative/democratic	This style is one where the leader values the input from their employees and uses input to make decisions. This is quite effective in boosting the morale of employees since they are part of the decision process. Changes are more easily accepted with this style due to the level of employee involvement
Transactional	In this style there is a reward for completion of a goal. Employees are given rewards or punishments based on the outcome of a task. The manager sets the goals with the employees, reviews their performances, and then decides on the reward or punishment
Transformational	The style of leadership is one in which the leader coaches and mentors his employees to make them better performers and better managers. Employees are motivated through good communication and positive coaching from the leader. This is effective when the leader is planning for future leaders or their eventual replacement
Charismatic	This type of leadership is one in which the leader uses their personality and charm to motivate and encourage employees to complete their tasks. The leader normally uses a lot of enthusiasm and positive feedback to direct their employees to success

non-owners of the corporation. Not-for-profit companies will have the board of trustees made up of individuals from the community along with the CEO of the organization.

Establishment of Mission, Vision, and Goals

The mission, vision, and goals of the organization define the reason the business exists, the direction the business wants to go, and the roles of key players who will accomplish these goals.

Mission—The mission is your statement that defines your existence. This statement reflects the beliefs about life, patients, practice, employees, and business objectives.

It serves as a guide to carry on business in a way defined by the core principles of the governance of the hospital. It should include some of the following:

Customers: Who are our customers?

Products or services: What are our products or services?

Markets: In what areas do we compete?

Concern for survival, growth, and profitability: What is our commitment toward economic strength and survivability?

Philosophy: What are our core beliefs, business philosophy, and values?

Concern for public image: What is our image in the community?

Concern for employees: What are our beliefs toward employees?

The mission statement can be very complex or very short. Here are a couple examples of mission statements:

The Ohio State University Wexner Medical Center: "to improve people's lives through innovation in research, education and patient care" (Medicalcenter.osu.edu 2013).

Akron Children's Hospital: "Akron Children's Hospital is dedicated to providing:

- Medical care to infants, children, adolescents and burn victims of all ages, regardless of ability to pay.
- Multi-level professional education for residents and students of medicine, nursing, and the various allied health professions.
- Basic and clinical research into the causes, treatment and cure of childhood illness and injury and burn injury.
- Community service intended to improve health status through lay education.
- Child and family advocacy efforts to improve the status of children and adolescents in our region of service.
- Continuing medical education to facilitate and encourage the process of lifelong learning for physicians and other health care providers involved in the care of children" (Akronchildrens.org 2013).

Duke University Hospital: "To provide exceptional and innovative care to patients, families, and the community through the finest integration of clinical care, education, and research while respecting the needs of the human spirit" (Dukehealth. org 2013).

Vision

The vision statement is a view of the company looking at where it wants to operate in the world and how it will operate. This should be a clear statement that is motivating and inspiring to those who read it and should convey the direction of the organization. The value of the statement is to provide high-level direction that the company will live by. It further defines your vision and mission and reflects the values of your organization. Some of the headings of the high statements include integrity, trust, ethics, quality, respect, healing, excellence, and teamwork.

Some examples of company's visions are:

The Ohio State University Wexner Medical Center: "working as a team, we will shape the future of medicine by creating, disseminating and applying new knowledge, and by personalizing health care to meet the needs of each individual" (Medicalcenter.osu.edu 2013).

Ann & Robert H. Lurie Children's Hospital of Chicago: "We are guided by the belief that all children need to grow up in a protective and nurturing environment where each child is given the opportunity to reach their full potential. We believe this vision can provide a brighter future for all children." "Our vision is inspired by the courage of children and families. It is sustained by the extraordinary contributions of compassionate, knowledgeable and dedicated staff and volunteers, and built from our tradition of providing unsurpassed health care for children dating back to 1882" (Luriechildrens.org 2013).

Duke University Hospital: "To be the recognized leader in patient and family-centered care, providing the finest environment for clinical education, improving the health of our community through clinical research, collaborative work culture that brings out the best in each of us, and supporting and investing in our community" (Dukehealth.org 2013).

Goals—Goals set by the governance of a health provider are tangible, well-thought-out strategic goals that your organization wishes to accomplish. A couple of goals could be:

- Perform financially to have 4 % operating margin.
- Use state-of-the-art medical technology to treat patients in the community.
- Coordinate comprehensive medical social services for the life of our patients.
- Maintain active partnerships with community and government services.

Governance Structure—The governance structure of an organization includes the bylaws of the organization and the structure of the authority in the organization. The bylaws of the company are the rules by which it operates as a business. These include both business and medical rules of operation for the business. The structure of authority in the organization is normally demonstrated by an organizational chart. Organizational charts start at the top with the board of trustees or board of directors and step down to the CEO and/or president at the second level of the chart. The next level of the chart will be the COO, CFO, and CMO. Following the third level of the chart is normally the vice president of the organization and then a split out of their divisions and subordinates in the next levels down. Below is a sample organization chart (Fig. 2.1).

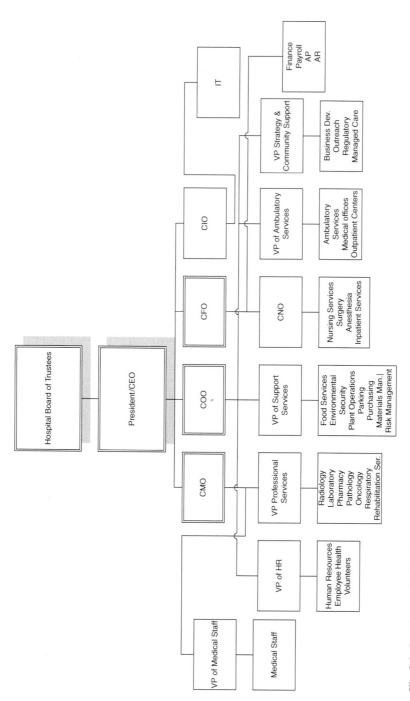

Fig. 2.1 Sample organization chart

Titles

There can be many different titles of administrators in the hospital, doctor's office, or other business. Below are some titles with their definitions:

Chairman of the board—The highest officer of the corporate board of directors or board of trustees.

Chief executive officer (CEO)—The top-ranking position in the company. The CEO can also hold the title of president.

President—Legally recognized highest corporate officer of the firm. If a company has both a CEO and a president, then the president will be the second highest-ranking officer in the organization.

Chief operating officer (COO)—This person answers directly to the CEO of the organization and is responsible for the overall operations of the business.

Chief financial officer (CFO)—This individual also answers directly to the CEO of the organization and is responsible for the corporate finances of the company.

Chief medical officer (CMO)—Answers to the CEO of the organization and is responsible for the medical staff of physicians in the organization.

Chief information officer (CIO)—Individual responsible for the information technology and all related operations.

Chief medical information officer (CMIO)—Individual responsible for the information technology dealing with any medical information and data in the hospital including electrical medical records.

Chief compliance officer (CCO)—Corporate official in charge of overseeing the management of compliance with issues within an organization.

Chief nursing officer (CNO)—individual responsible for all divisions within the hospital in which nursing is involved, normally answers to the COO.

VP—Middle or upper manager of the corporation, normally answers directly to the COO, CFO, or CMO and is normally responsible for a range of departments in the organization.

Director—Individual that has different departments of an organization, such as the director of nursing.

There are many other titles, terms, and acronyms used in business than those mentioned here. The majority of the upper-level management positions are normally included in these titles. One should be familiar with these different titles and their duties in order to properly operate in an organization.

The goal of this chapter was to define the leadership and governance as it may appear in different types of organizations. All businesses need leaders and structure in order to be successful, to be compliant with authorities, and to complete the purpose the business was created for. This chapter has laid the groundwork of how organizations are set up, operated, and managed. The balance of the text will be introducing knowledge, tools, skills, and explanations of how a physician or a non-physician can operate in an administrative position in a healthcare setting. Some of these tools will be financial such as the financial statements of the organization, while some will be explanations and descriptions of different pieces and parts of the healthcare business such as insurance, managed care, and the future of healthcare in the country.

Further Reading

Akronchildrens.org. Mission: Akron Children's Hospital. (Online) https://www.akronchildrens. org/cms/hospital_mission_and_commitment/index.html (2013). Accessed 9 Oct 2013.

Barton P. Understanding the U.S. health services system. Chicago, IL: Health Administration Press; 2010.

Buchbinder S, Shanks N. Introduction to health care management. Burlington, MA: Jones & Bartlett Learning; 2012.

Dahl O. Think business! Phoenix, MD: Greenbranch; 2007.

Dukehealth.org. Mission, vision, and values – Duke University Hospital – DukeHealth.org. (Online) http://www.dukehealth.org/locations/duke_hospital/location_details/duke_university_hospital_mission (2013). Accessed 9 Oct 2013.

Fallon L, Mcconnell C (in press) Human resource management in health care.

Keagy B, Thomas M. Essentials of physician practice management. San Francisco: Jossey-Bass; 2004.

Luriechildrens.org. Vision & mission, Children's Hospital – Lurie Children's. (Online) https://www.luriechildrens.org/en-us/about-us/Pages/vision-mission.aspx (2013). Accessed 9 Oct 2013.

Marcinko D, Hetico H. The business of medical practice. New York: Springer; 2011.

Mcconnell C, Umiker W. Umiker's management skills for the new health care supervisor. Burlington, MA: Jones & Bartlett Learning; 2014.

Medicalcenter.osu.edu. About us. (Online) http://medicalcenter.osu.edu/aboutus/Pages/index.aspx (2013). Accessed 9 Oct 2013.

Niles N. Basics of the U.S. health care system. Sudbury, MA: Jones and Bartlett; 2011.

Rubino L, Esparza S, Chassiakos Y. New leadership for today's health care professionals. Burlington, MA: Jones & Bartlett Learning; 2014.

Shi L, Singh D. Delivering health care in America. Sudbury, MA: Jones & Bartlett Learning; 2012.

Shi L, Singh D. Essentials of the U.S. health care system. Burlington, MA: Jones & Bartlett Learning; 2013.

Solomon R. The physician manager's handbook. Sudbury, MA: Jones and Bartlett; 2008.

Sultz H, Young K. Health care USA. Burlington, MA: Jones & Bartlett Learning; 2014.

Yousem D, Beauchamp N. Radiology business practice. Philadelphia: Saunders/Elsevier; 2008.

Chapter 3
Revenue Cycle

Abstract The revenue cycle is the entire medical billing process from the beginning to the end. It would include the entire cycle of a patient medical service from scheduling to payment and consists of the administrative and clinical functions that are part of the capture, management, and collection of patient revenue. A properly working revenue cycle is very important to the financial success of a business. This process is a cycle because it is repeated every time a patient has a different service. The revenue cycle consists of scheduling the patient, the registration, and the medical service provided, capturing the charges for the visit, processing the bills, and finally collecting the revenue. Most services in the medical business are provided on credit since most patients have some type of insurance or third-party support to pay for their medical expenses. With this type of payment for service, the revenue cycle is a process for which we document, verify, bill, and collect for services rendered. This revenue cycle can make or break a business financially. Any malfunctions or errors in any step of the revenue cycle can delay the payment services, deny the payment, or cause the office to rework the revenue cycle and resubmit more information for services. The goal of any medical business should be to have the revenue cycle operating efficiently and effectively to collect revenue for the service provided. With the collection of revenues from the revenue cycle comes cash in other certificates of monetary value that needs to be safeguarded and secured. A system needs to be established for the protection of the revenue collected from this revenue cycle.

The revenue cycle is composed of eight integrated and overlapping steps. Figure 3.1 shows the revenue cycle to be described in this chapter. Each part is as important as the others:

- Scheduling
- Registration/authorization
- Clinical services
- Charge capture
- Claims processing

R.V. Bucci, *Medicine and Business: A Practitioner's Guide*,
DOI 10.1007/978-3-319-04060-8_3, © Springer International Publishing Switzerland 2014

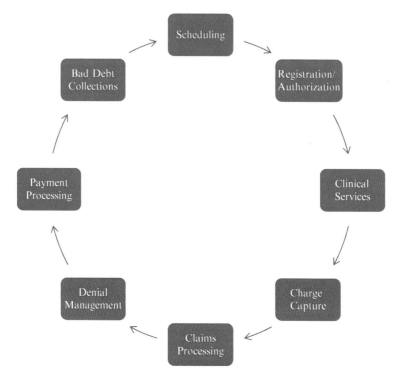

Fig. 3.1 Revenue cycle

- Denial management
- Payment processing
- Bad debt and collections

Revenue Cycle Steps

Scheduling

Scheduling the patient for a service is the first step of the revenue cycle. The scheduling department of a medical business can be seen as a front door of the business. This is normally the first interaction of a patient with a medical provider and is your patient's first impression of how your medical business runs.

The scheduling portion of a business can be of different sizes and structure. In small businesses, it can be one person, but as a practice gets larger, more staff is required. As the size of the business grows, a scheduling department may be needed. In health systems or hospital systems, scheduling is performed either by each department for their own services or by a central scheduling department that schedules for all departments. There are positives and negatives for each type of scheduling structure which need to be evaluated on a case-by-case basis.

Scheduling can occur in a number of ways as well. Traditionally, scheduling has always been accomplished via a telephone call. Technology, however, has changed how scheduling can occur. Patients are now able to schedule their appointments online interactively with their computers, phones, or tablet devices. The medical business should be prepared to offer all types of scheduling in order to stay competitive.

The key function of the scheduler is to balance the needs of the patients with the needs of the medical practice. The scheduler should accommodate the patients' needs, wants, and desires by giving them the appropriate appointment, thus giving them a good patient experience. The goal for a scheduler is to accommodate the maximum amount of patients in a given workday to maximize the facility revenue. Unfilled appointments mean a loss of revenue for the practice. Some of the keys to successful scheduling are as follows:

- Schedule all open appointments.
- Schedule the appropriate procedures or visits during the appropriate times and resources. The patient which is scheduled in the wrong time or place for their service will cause rescheduling, loss of revenue, and dissatisfaction of the patient.
- Schedule enough time to accommodate the patient service. If not enough time is scheduled for a patient visit, then backups and rescheduling of visits can also occur.
- Keep a cancelation list or move up list. Cancelations are inevitable. You should have a list of patients willing to move up with short notice to fill these appointments.
- Reminder calls. Patients should be called the day or two days before their scheduled appointment to verify that they will be coming in for that appointment.
- Leave a couple openings in the schedule to accommodate emergencies and walk-ins.
- Be flexible with patients in office schedules. One should always work with both the patients and the office schedules to maximize patient satisfaction and business revenue.

Registration/Authorization

This is the second part of the revenue cycle and can be considered the most important part. Registration can occur prior to coming in for the appointment, at the appointment, or a mixture of the two. Registration includes gathering important information regarding the patient's demographic information including their address, telephone number, and place of work and the insurance coverage information. Any inaccurate information in any of these areas will cause delays or nonpayment of services rendered to the patient. If a patient's insurance identification number is incorrectly recorded, the insurance company will not pay the bill, but will be returned to the business.

The second part of registration includes authorization of services. Many services have to be preapproved or authorized before the patient can have the service. A patient having an MRI scan may need approval by the insurance company to guarantee that the exam is allowed and will be paid. This is a normal process for most services that are of high reimbursement amounts. If a medical office performs services without preapproval when preapproval was required, then the services will not be paid for by the insurance company. If the services are denied for no approval by the insurance company, then the responsibility for payment will fall on the patient. This situation can cause a financial hardship to the patient and a negative impression of the business. For government payers such as Medicare and Medicaid, if preapproval is not obtained for a service, then the service will not be paid for by them and the patient will not be held responsible for the payment either. The medical business will have to write off the entire bill.

The registration and authorization sections of the revenue cycle are vital to the cash flow of a medical business. Obtaining accurate information and necessary authorizations is key to success in this part of the revenue cycle.

Clinical Services

Clinical services are the actual medical services performed, whether it is an office visit, test, hospital stay, and so forth. All staff should make this a pleasant experience for the patient while performing high-quality medical care. During this time, proper and accurate documentation of all services performed on a patient is essential to the revenue cycle. All clinical procedure and services occurring during the patient visit needs to be documented or it may not be paid for by the insurance company.

Charge Capture

Charge capture is the transfer of the documented information from the clinical visit to the medical records and billing system. Services that are procedures performed at the visit need to be assigned a CPT code and an ICD-9 code. A CPT code is a five-digit number assigned to every service performed for patients including lab exams, office visits, and surgeries. A typical office visit may have a CPT code of 99211 or a flu shot will have a code of 90658. An ICD-9 code is a numerical code that specifies a disease or diagnosis. Typical codes are 782.3 for edema or swelling and 486 for pneumonia. A proper charge capture includes both the ICD-9 and the CPT codes matched together in regard to the diagnosis of the patient and a procedure completed. If these two codes do not match up in regard to medical and logical sense, then the claim may be denied or returned for inaccurate billing. It is important to verify that these codes match in the documentation completed during the clinical visit.

A second aspect of charge capture is to match the ICD-9 code and CPT code to the preauthorization information. If a patient was approved to have an MRI scan by the insurance company, then the CPT and ICD-9 codes which were approved must be used for billing purposes. If this medical facility would bill an insurance carrier with different ICD-9 or CPT codes than were approved, then the claim will probably not be paid.

Claims Processing

The next step in the process is to submit the claims or bills out to the insurance companies and/or patients. The majority of medical service companies have some type of electronic billing system, while some companies still use paper claims and statements to get paid for their services. The claims processing part of the medical business needs to transfer the charge capture information onto a claims form required for the individual insurance company or payer and then transfer that claims information to that payer. Most payers accept the CMS-1450, which was formally called the UB-92, which is designed for hospitals and skilled nursing and home healthcare facilities. For physicians and outpatient services, the CMS-1500 form, formerly the HCFA-1500 form, is used for the billing of services rendered at your facility.

If the patient is paying for the service themselves or after the patient's insurance company has paid their portion of the bill, the company will send a statement of services to the patient for payment. The patient will be responsible for paying their portion of the bill. An efficient billing division or company will be diligent in managing these claims for proper payment of services received.

Denial Management

After the insurance company or other payer receives the claims from the medical provider, they may deny all or a portion of the claims. The reasons for denials can be inaccurate CPT or ICD-9 codes, incorrect information in patient demographics such as the patient's name and address, or incorrect insurance identification numbers. There are many reasons that denials occur. This is the most frustrating part of the revenue cycle because the medical office will have to spend time to research the denial and then submit corrections or justifications.

This is a labor-intensive part of the business, but it must be completed in order to capture all the revenue that was earned by the service.

Payment Processing

After payments are received from either the insurance company or the patient, then the payments must be entered into the billing system. Insurance companies pay via a check or wire transfer. When insurance pays, there is normally an adjustable or contractually discounted amount to be reduced from the patient's bill. A patient's bill for services may be $100.00 for a certain procedure. The medical business may have a contract with the insurance company that states that this service will be paid for at $65.00. Then the remaining $35.00 will be deducted as a contractual discount. Co-payments and contractual adjustments will be discussed extensively in a later chapter. This will be the last step in the revenue cycle if the patient's balance is $0.0 after payments and contractual discounts by the insurance company and/or the patient. If all steps to collect internally are exhausted and the balance is not $0.0, then the next step will apply.

Bad Debt and Collections

This step occurs when payment for services rendered is not received in a predetermined amount of time. The medical provider will bill for services as designated in the previous steps of the revenue cycle. If the payment is not received in a certain amount of time and the provider feels that it has exhausted all of its efforts to collect payments for the services, then they have two options. The first option is bad debt write-off. This is where the provider will just write off or discount from the bill the amount not paid by the patient or the insurance company. The other option is to turn the patient over to a third-party collection agency. This should be the last step in collections since it can harm provider-patient relationships. The collection agency will then use its best efforts to collect the money from the responsible party. Both of these options are revenue losses to the corporation. While bad debt loses all of the money due, the collection agency will normally give the business two thirds of the collections and keep one third for collecting the debt.

Revenue Cycle Options and Monitoring

Items to address in the revenue cycle include decisions of whether to keep the billing inside your company (internal) or to outsource (external) it to a professional billing company and which key indicators of financial performance metrics need to be used in monitoring the revenue cycle.

Key Indicators

Once the revenue cycle is up and running, there is a need to analyze the revenue cycle for its efficiency and ability to collect payments. There are some financial tools that will help us analyze the system. The key financial trackers of the revenue cycle will be discussed briefly below and more in Chap. 8 of this text:

- *Days in accounts receivable*—The average time it takes to collect payment for the procedure or service after it was performed.
- *Days cash on hand*—The number of days of expenses that the current firm can pay with cash on hand at today's cash collection rate, a percentage of the cash collected in regard to the net revenue for the same period of time.
- *Bad debt write-off*—The amount of bad debt you write off in comparison to the gross revenue.
- *The cost to collect*—It's a total of the business office expenses divided by the cash collections achieved with these resources.
- *An aging schedule*—Breakdown that shows the firm accounts receivable by 30, 60, 90, and over 120 days.

Accounts Payable In-House or Outsourcing—Accounts payable, coding, and claims processing can be completed by the medical businesses' employees or contracted out to outside billing companies. The correct decision depends on the age of the business, size of the medical company, level of knowledge of coding and billing of the company staff, and the amount of information technology or computer systems. There is no true formula for whether a company should outsource or keep in-house. Some of the pros and cons are:

Internal billing:

Pros

> Control over employees, procedures, and financial operations
> Proximity of billing department
> Transparency

Cons

> Higher expenses
> Finding, training, and retaining knowledgeable staff
> Administrative burdens

External billing:

Pros

> Less capital investment in billing software and computer hardware
> More personnel and support
> Personnel are updated on regulation and coding changes
> Lower billing costs

Cons

> Loss of control
> Possible loss of quality
> Low dollar claims may not receive adequate treatment.
> Risk of fraud.
> Hidden fees.

Internal Safeguards and Controls

The purpose of the revenue cycle is to bill and collect for the provision of healthcare services. This revenue is used to pay for the expenses of the business, growth of the business, and shareholder profits or community investment, depending on the type of business. The revenue will enter the business in different forms including cash, personal business checks, money orders, or direct deposit to a bank account. These instruments of value, especially cash, need to be protected against loss, theft, or possible embezzlement. Whenever there is cash involved in the business, there's always the possibility of loss in some manner. Every business should set up some type of internal controls or check-and-balance system in order to keep its collected revenues safe.

Internal Cash Controls

The inappropriate or unauthorized use of company funds can occur in any business. Every business that deals with cash and cash equivalents should set up internal cash controls to protect its business from theft, embezzlements, and fraud. These controls will also have the positive effect of increasing the accuracy and reliability of accounting records. Internal controls are actually required for all publically traded US corporations under the authority of the Sarbanes-Oxley Act of 2002. It is simply smart business for every other business. Some steps to protect the firm are to establish responsibilities, segregate duties, reconciliation, and securing your money.

Funds Entering the Business

There are a number of ways in which payments can enter a medical practice during any given day:

- Cash, checks, and money orders received through the mail from patients and third-party payers
- Payments received in person from patients directly at the office or healthcare facility
- Credit or debit card payment received in person, over the phone, or by mail
- Funds directly deposited into the healthcare business banking accounts

Internal controls are policies and procedures applied to collecting, documenting, and securing inflows of funds into the business. These controls should be tailored to the business so that they are practical, realistic, and attainable for the business. With these policies will come expectations for accurate documentation and verification of all steps involved from collecting the cash to the time it is deposited into a bank account.

Establish Responsibilities—Only specific individuals should be assigned to the responsibilities of collecting the cash, recording the transaction, and storing the funds. Control is gained by having fewer people involved in the receipt of money.

Segregation of Duties—Different parts of a cash transaction should be assigned to different individuals. Different individuals should receive cash, record cash receipts, and secure the cash. The person opening the mail or taking payments should not be the same person that is posting these payments against the patient accounts. These roles should rotate periodically as a safety measure. Procedures for handling cash should be clearly defined and understood by all staff members.

Documentation of Receipts—The following information is necessary to audit, verify, and accurately record all payments:

- The person who took the payment
- The amount of payment received
- To whom the payment is or should be applied to
- Type of payment in regard to insurance check, personal check, cash, credit card, or money order
- The totals of each type of payment
- The date and time and location of the payment
- How the payment was received

Reconciliation—Funds that come into a medical practice can be for current services, future services, and previous services. These receipts should be reconciled daily against the medical billing records of the patients along with the remittance receipts or deposit slips. This reconciliation should be completed by someone else rather than the person receiving the payments.

Security of Cash Receipts—Funds should be secured in the office until delivered to a banking account. These funds should be stored in a secure location such as a safe or locked storage cabinet. The cash and checks should be delivered to a bank on a daily basis to reduce the amount of cash on hand.

Warning Signs of Unauthorized Use of Funds

Fraud, embezzlement, and theft are all terms for misappropriation of funds. This can be a problem in a medical business, as well as any other business. These problems usually happen due to lack of internal controls, allowing somebody in the office to have too many responsibilities or having individuals with too much authority. Some possible instances of misappropriation of funds are as follows:

- Receiving a patient's payment and not turning it into the business.
- Skimming a portion of a patient's payment for themselves and turning a portion of it into the business. A patient may pay $25 in cash and they will turn into $20 to business and keep the other $5 for themselves.
- Receiving the patient's payment for services and recording it in the accounts receivable as a write-off. They then take the full amount of cash.
- Taking money from the petty cash account.

- Using the company's funds or checking account to pay personal liabilities and bills.
- Stealing a patient's check or money order and forging the signature.
- Purchasing products or supplies with company funds and taking those products home.
- Billing schemes that create fictitious bills for patients and then keeping the money that is paid for them.
- When an account is overpaid by a patient or an insurance company, they can take that money and not refund the overpayment.
- Creating fictitious expenses that the business will pay and the employee will steal the funds.
- Temporarily borrowing practice funds with the intent to pay them back later. The payback may or may not occur.
- Stealing miscellaneous income money that is not recorded. This can include income from fees for copies of records, filling out documents, or other fictitious charges.
- Erroneous or fraudulent invoices approved for payment.
- Unauthorized payments made to nonexistent vendors.

Tips to Internal Control

- Set up written policies and procedures to make sure all employees adhere to them.
- Open a lockbox for payments to be received directly as opposed to delivered to the office.
- Stamp checks for "deposit only" for the company as they enter the business.
- Bank deposit should be made on a regular or daily basis. There should be a separate deposit for each day's receipts, even if the deposit is not taken to the bank on a daily basis.
- Insurance checks and their explanation of benefits statement should be reviewed and verified for accuracy.
- Individual payments and checks should be listed separately on the deposit slips to serve as an audit trail for reconciliation.
- Any money received for items other than the patient accounts such as rental incomes, physician honorariums, or other services outside of the medical practice should be deposited separately from the patient account deposits.
- Someone outside of the business such as an accountant or CPA should perform regularly scheduled audits and bank reconciliations as a good safety measure.
- It is a good idea to have all employees handling cash be "bonded." Bonding is a type of insurance protection that covers theft or dishonesty of employees in the business.

Petty Cash

Most businesses set up a petty cash account that should be $100 or less to pay for small expenses of the business that may be impractical or unable to be paid by a check. Items purchased with a petty cash account are small items from office supply stores or grocery stores, postage money, or expenses of the business that are of low amounts. There should be petty cash policy for these disbursements so that this money does not go missing.

- The administrator should approve all the purchases using petty cash.
- Petty cash funds should be counted, balanced, and reconciled daily by a second assigned person in the office.
- Receipts should be written for all dispersed petty cash.
- Receipts of purchases should be attached to the receipts of the disbursements.
- Petty cash funds should not be used as a bank source for personal checks or IOUs.

Bank Accounts

Healthcare businesses need to establish bank accounts to manage their money from the business. A couple of different types of accounts should be formed for every business:

Business checking account—A regular checking account should be established to receive money from patient services and to be used for disbursements of expenses and payroll. This is normally the regular business checking account. There should be sufficient funds in the account to pay for outstanding checks and payroll.

Money market for sweep investment account—This is an interest-generating account that can earn additional money for the business. The sweep account generally takes money from the checking account over a set minimum amount and then deposits it in an interest-bearing account such as a money market account. This is an automatic transaction that can take place when decided by the business such as everyday or once per week. This is generally a good idea since the checking account normally does not bear interest.

Lockbox account—A lockbox account is a smart way to have the deposits from your business sent directly to your banking account. When billing insurance companies and patients for services rendered, the remittance address can be that of the bank lockbox. All payments for the business will be sent to this lockbox which directly deposits all funds into your business checking account. This eliminates the cast majority of money physically coming into your business and makes it much more secure. The lockbox normally has features to notify you daily with deposit information including amounts and receipts.

Control of Expense Payments

Fraud can occur on the payment of expense side of the business just as easy as the income of cash and the business. Many of the same rules applied to the intake of money into the business will apply to this outflow including:

Establish responsibilities—Only specific individuals should be assigned to the payment of expenses and payroll. A specific set of individuals should be responsible for the payment of expenses of the business, documentation, and verification of all paid expenses.

Segregation of duties—Different parts of a cash transaction should be assigned to different individuals. Different individuals should authorize the bills or invoices and write the actual checks. These roles should rotate periodically as a safety measure. Procedures for paying accounts payable should be clearly defined and understood by all staff members.

Reconciliation—Payments for accounts payable should be reconciled against the company checking account and the matching invoices or bills. This reconciliation should be performed by a person other than the person writing the checks for the bills. The accountant should also reconcile the banking account against the records of the bills. Some best practices include:

• Review vendor invoices for accuracy by comparing charges to purchase orders.
• Verify that the goods and services purchased have been received.
• Perform monthly reconciliations of operating ledgers to assure accuracy and timeliness of expenses.

Signing of checks—The authorization or signing of checks should be signed by two people. One person should be the custodian in charge of writing the checks for the bills, and the other should be the president or other high-ranking officer of the business to verify and sign off on all bills and invoices.

Summary

The revenue cycle is a complete cycle of the patient medical series from the scheduling of the patient until the patient account is paid or written off. Accurate documentation, coding, and billing are essential to the healthcare business's financial survival. A well-run revenue cycle in a business can make or break the company financially.

Now that we have seen how a medical company receives revenues for services, the next four chapters will focus on how to look at the revenues and expenses of the business in the form of financial statements and ratios for an analysis of the business.

Further Reading

Cleverley W, Cleverley J, Song P. Essentials of health care finance. Sudbury, MA: Jones & Bartlett Learning; 2011.

Finkler S, Ward D. Accounting fundamentals for health care management. Sudbury, MA: Jones and Bartlett; 2006.

Gapenski L, Pink G. Understanding healthcare financial management. Chicago: Health Administration Press; 2011.

Getzen T. Health economics and financing. Hoboken, NJ: Wiley; 2010.

Getzen T. Health economics and financing. Hoboken: Wiley; 2013.

Huss W, Coleman M. Start your own medical practice. Naperville, IL: Sphinx; 2006.

Keagy B, Thomas M. Essentials of physician practice management. San Francisco: Jossey-Bass; 2004.

Kongstvedt P. Managed care. Boston: Jones and Bartlett; 2004.

Marcinko D, Hetico H. The business of medical practice. New York: Springer; 2011.

Reiboldt J. Financial management of the medical practice. Chicago, IL: American Medical Association; 2011.

Solomon R. The physician manager's handbook. Sudbury, MA: Jones and Bartlett; 2008.

Yousem D, Beauchamp N. Radiology business practice. Philadelphia: Saunders/Elsevier; 2008.

Chapter 4
Financial Definitions and Variances

Abstract This chapter will review some of the financial and accounting definitions and terms that will be used throughout this book in the financial area. There are many variables in the accounting and reporting world that you need to be aware of when reviewing and analyzing financial information. Some differences in accounting techniques will determine if a patient's service is added to the financial books of the company when it occurs at a point in time later. This will also affect the report you generate from the records. Services performed in a particular day can be posted to the financial books either on the same day the services were performed or at a date later than the actual day of service. Some different accounting terminology and account principles will be explained including cash basis accounting versus accrual basis accounting, variable and fixed costs, posting by date of service versus by date of such posting, etc. General definitions and assumptions of accounting will also be defined in this chapter. A general knowledge of these definitions is required so that you are able to understand the financial statements of your organization.

Definitions

Accounting Entity—The entity is the business to which the financial statements pertain. This is important when reviewing the financial statements of a large hospital system with many entities. Each individual entity may have their own set of financial statements, and then these statements are rolled up into one consolidated financial statement. Therefore, one must be careful when determining which entity the financial data belongs to.

Going Concern—This means that one assumes that the company will operate indefinitely into the future. This principle is useful when determining such things as a basis for the value of assets in the company. The valuation of the business and its parts is based on the philosophy that the business will keep running indefinitely.

R.V. Bucci, *Medicine and Business: A Practitioner's Guide*,
DOI 10.1007/978-3-319-04060-8_4, © Springer International Publishing Switzerland 2014

Accounting Period—This is the amount of time that the income statement represents, such as a month or a year. Many companies use the calendar year as the fiscal year, but some companies' fiscal year may vary, such as October 1 to September 30.

Monetary Units—This is simply the unit or currency in which transactions are represented. In the United States, for example, the monetary unit would be the dollar.

Historical Costs—This is a principle that requires organizations to report the values of their assets on acquisition costs rather than fair market value. For example, a building purchased 10 years ago for $100,000 may be worth $1 million today in fair market value but is still reported on the books as $100,000.

Revenue Recognition—This principle requires that revenues are recognized in the same period in which they are earned and realized. For example, an MRI procedure that was completed in December would be recorded on the books as December revenue, whether payment for the procedure was received in December or not.

Cost Matching—This principle requires organizations to match revenues and related expenses. In other words, after revenues for a certain period are recognized, the expenses that have been associated with those revenues should be accounted for in the same period.

Full Disclosure—The financial statements of an entity must show a complete picture of all economic events and transactions of the business. If all economic events are not included, the financial statements would be misleading and not represent the company's true financial picture.

Objectivity—A constraint of the financial documents is there must be objective and verifiable supporting data and documentation for all of the transactions reported in the statements. This verification and documentation can be in the form of things such as patient bills, invoices, and bank statements.

Consistency—This involves the company using similar guidelines to report different transactions over time. Using the same methods and procedures to collect and report data gives credibility to the statements and allows the company to accurately track performance trends. Essentially, consistency in this area guarantees that you're comparing apples to apples and oranges to oranges.

Conservatism—This is a principle that constrains the firm to record financial information in a way that will least likely overstate the business's financial condition. Accounting methods should always choose the path that will least likely overstate the company's condition.

Depreciation and Amortization—In accrual accounting, we need some way of recognizing assets on the financial statements. We look at an asset such as a piece of equipment, building, or a patent, and we determine the length of service or life we will get out of that asset. For example, we purchase a CT scanner and expect to use it in the hospital for 7 years before we replace it. We would say the CT scanner has an expected useful life of 7 years. Now, we need to expense that CT scanner over 7 years. If the purchase price was $700,000, then we would expense $100,000 per year in the depreciation and amortization section of the income statement. This would also be reflected in the balance sheet in the statement of cash flow.

The difference between depreciation and amortization is the type of assets represented. Depreciation refers to assets that are real or tangible such as machines, land, and buildings. Amortization is the term referred to when expanding the life of intangible or untouchable types of assets such as goodwill, patents, and trademarks. Many times these will be reported on the same expense line of the operating income statement. They can be reflected in a number of ways on the balance sheet, but they will always be in the fixed asset section.

Variances

Cash Basis Versus Accrual Accounting

There are two ways to look at accounting in regard to how transactions are entered and accounted for. These methods will impact your monthly financial statements, your monthly reports, and your taxes.

Cash Basis Accounting—Cash basis accounting is when you recognize or post revenues and expenses when there is actual cash transacted. This means that the only time that any kind of activity gets accounted for is when cash actually moves from one company or individual to another company or individual. A person may have a medical procedure or test in October which is not paid for until November. In cash basis accounting, that event would be recorded in November, when the actual cash was received. The transaction is posted when the actual cash is paid to the vendor as opposed to when the invoice or product was received or used.

Accrual Accounting—Accrual-based accounting is when you recognize or post expenses and revenues when they occur rather than when the cash changes hands. This method records economic events when a transaction takes place rather than when the payment is actually received. A person may have a medical procedure in October which is not paid for until November. In accrual-based accounting, this event would be recorded in October when the treatment was received. This type of accounting also records expenses associated with a service at the time the service was rendered.

An advantage of the cash basis is that the inflated accounts receivable are not recognized for tax purposes, while a disadvantage is that cash basis does not show a true picture of your firm's financial status. Accrual-based accounting shows a more accurate status of your financial position and is used by most larger firms. It is the choice not only because it shows greater accuracy but also because it provides an easy way to consolidate statements from multiple divisions.

Date of Posting Versus Date of Service

Date of Service—Another variant in reporting of activity in the healthcare business would be if services are recorded by date of posting or date of service. If the activities are posted by date of service, then you will see an activity registered in the books on the actual date it was performed. If it is recorded by date of posting, this will occur either on the day of service or sometime in the future. Learning the difference between these two will help you review and analyze reports more accurately. An example of an MRI center will show the difference. In the months of January, February, and March, there were 200, 150, and 180 MRI scans performed, respectively. For simplicity, the cost of each scan is $1,000.

The chart below shows how these MRI scans would be reported utilizing the date of service method. This method is fairly straightforward.

Month	Jan	Feb	Mar
MRI scans	200	150	180
Charges	$200,000	$150,000	$180,000

Date of Posting—In reality, charges for services rendered are not posted to the books on the date of service. Most hospitals hold charges at least 3 days in order to collect financial data, document results, and obtain inpatient demographic information. Sometimes these factors take longer than 3 days to collect and posting is delayed even further. In the "date of posting" example below, the MRI scans performed in the last 3 days of January will not be recorded in the books until February. In this example, 25 scans were performe in December and the 150 scans were performe in January, but, they were all posted in January. February postings included two scans from December, 40 scans from January, and 90 from February. The posting for March included 10 from January, 35 from February, and 140 from March. You can see the differences in the totals compared to the above date of service postings.

Month	Jan	Feb	Mar
December	25	2	0
January	150	40	10
February		125	15
March			140
Total	$175,000	$167,000	$165,000

You have now seen that the financials can look completely different for the two different methods. This can also make a large impact when reviewing reports on a monthly basis. One has to determine if the reports should be based on date of service or date of posting. For example, when reviewing the number of MRI scans completed on a monthly basis for a trend, it would be best to review these on a date of service method so that you can view the actual number of scans completed that month.

Expenses: Fixed Versus Variable Cost and Direct Versus Indirect Costs

Expenses can be broken down into two sets of categories. One category consists of fixed costs versus variable costs, and the second category deals with direct versus indirect costs.

Fixed Costs—A fixed cost can be an expense such as the rent, the malpractice insurance, or the phone bill charge. These expenses will occur whether or not you conduct any business and they must be paid. Whether your firm has 0 patients in the month or 500, the fixed costs will remain constant and will need to be paid.

Variable Costs—The other type of expense is a variable cost. Examples of variable costs are splints, contrast for radiology procedures, or prescription drugs given to a patient. These expenses fluctuate with the volume of services provided. They are only incurred if you use them for a patient. If you do not use them, then no costs are incurred. Labor costs can be divided as well. A salary paid to a person such as a manager could be considered a fixed cost since their salary will be paid the same each pay period. An hourly worker, on the other hand, could be considered variable if they only work when needed.

Direct Costs—A direct cost describes something directly related to taking care of the patient. This could describe the medical supplies used during the case, the cost of the nurse, and the medical equipment used for the patient. These costs are directly related to patient care and are specific to the service being performed.

Indirect Cost—An indirect cost is not related to the care of a patient. These can be the cost of the cable TV in the lobby, office rent, salaries of the billing staff, or the cost of building insurance. These are costs that are more general to the business and not directly associated with the care of a patient. When reviewing expenses to be decreased for cost containment, indirect expenses are the first ones to be reviewed.

Further Reading

Cleverley W, Cleverley J, Song P. Essentials of health care finance. Sudbury, MA: Jones & Bartlett Learning; 2011.

Finkler S, Ward D. Accounting fundamentals for health care management. Sudbury, MA: Jones and Bartlett; 2006.

Gapenski L, Pink G. Understanding healthcare financial management. Chicago, IL: Health Administration Press; 2011.

Getzen T. Health economics and financing. Hoboken, NJ: Wiley; 2010.

Getzen T. Health economics and financing. Hoboken, NJ: Wiley; 2013.

Huss W, Coleman M. Start your own medical practice. Naperville, IL: Sphinx; 2006.

Keagy B, Thomas M. Essentials of physician practice management. San Francisco, CA: Jossey-Bass; 2004.

Kongstvedt P. Managed care. Boston, MA: Jones and Bartlett; 2004.

Marcinko D, Hetico H. The business of medical practice. New York: Springer; 2011.

Reiboldt J. Financial management of the medical practice. Chicago, IL: American Medical Association; 2011.

Solomon R. The physician manager's handbook. Sudbury, MA: Jones and Bartlett; 2008.

Yousem D, Beauchamp N. Radiology business practice. Philadelphia, PA: Saunders/Elsevier; 2008.

Chapter 5
Income Statement

Abstract A company's financial statements are mathematical pictures which we use to determine the financial status of the company. The next three chapters will review the three key financial statements, including the income statement, the balance sheet, and the statement of cash flow. Whether you work for a small practice or a large hospital system, all businesses have financial statements which should be understood by those in decision-making positions. The first statement that we will look at is the income statement. The income statement is a view of the company's operations in terms of financial numbers over a time period such as a month or year. The income statement can be very basic with few line items or can be quite extensive for a large corporation such as a hospital. As we move through parts of the income statement, a simple statement will be built into a more complex statement. Each section will be discussed and then added to the income statement. For all financial statements, there is no standard template that all companies must use. Each company will design the layout of their statements as represented by their industry, profit status, and personal preferences.

This is probably the most important statement that you will have in the business because it tells you whether or not you are making a profit. There are many other names used to describe the income statement. Other names that can be used for the income statement are:

- Statement of operations
- Profit loss statement
- Statement of income and expenses
- Operating statement
- Activity statement

For the purposes of this book, it will be described as the income statement.

The basic parts of an income statement are income, expenses, and net income as shown in Fig. 5.1. The revenue and expenses can be broken down into different

R.V. Bucci, *Medicine and Business: A Practitioner's Guide*,   41
DOI 10.1007/978-3-319-04060-8_5, © Springer International Publishing Switzerland 2014

Buckeye Medical Center
Income Statement
Years Ending December 31, 2012 and 2011

Financial statements in U.S. dollars	2012	2011	Increase / (Decrease)	Percent Change
	(In Thousands)			
Operating Revenue				
Operating Revenue	1,109,822	958,874	150,948	15.74%
Less: Contractual Discounts	410,634	354,783	55,851	15.74%
Net Operating Revenue	699,188	604,091	95,097	15.74%
Operating Expenses				
Salaries and Wages - Non Physician	221,504	181,562	39,942	22.00%
Professional Fees	85,371	69,977	15,394	22.00%
Employee Benefits	89,986	73,759	16,227	22.00%
Supplies	69,220	56,738	12,482	22.00%
Purchased Services	48,454	39,716	8,738	22.00%
Facilities	29,995	24,586	5,409	22.00%
Insurance	11,536	9,456	2,080	22.00%
Utilities	9,229	7,565	1,664	22.00%
Interest Expense	8,625	7,902	723	9.15%
Depreciation and Amortization	41,532	34,042	7,490	22.00%
Bad Debt	13,599	15,599	(2,000)	-12.82%
Other	4,514	3,782	732	19.35%
Total Operating Expenses	633,565	524,684	108,881	20.75%
Income From Operations	65,623	79,407	(13,784)	-17.36%
Non Operating Revenue (Expenses)				
Investment Income (loss)	15,000	(12,500)	27,500	-220.00%
Community Support and Charity	(55,682)	(45,893)		
Other	7,596	8,569	(973)	-11.35%
Total Non Operating Incom e	(33,086)	(49,824)	16,738	-33.59%
Net Income (Loss)	32,537	29,583	2,954	9.99%

Buckeye Medical Center
Income Statement
Years Ending December 31, 2012 and 2011

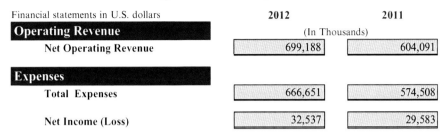

Financial statements in U.S. dollars	2012	2011
Operating Revenue	(In Thousands)	
Net Operating Revenue	699,188	604,091
Expenses		
Total Expenses	666,651	574,508
Net Income (Loss)	32,537	29,583

Fig. 5.1 Basics Parts of Income Statement. Operating Income less Expenses Equals Net income

parts. The basic equation for the income statement is income minus expenses equals net revenue is:

$$Operating\ Income - Expenses = Net\ Income$$

Revenue

Operating Revenue or Medical Services Revenue

Operating revenue and medical services revenue are terms that can be inter-changed and are the revenue that you receive from performing services on patients, such as office visits, medical tests, patient hospital days, or surgeries. The revenue for all services provided is normally presented as one line item and includes all of the medical services provided in that institution. Normally, a busi-ness in healthcare reports their income statement according to the accrual basis. With accrual accounting, you record all transactions when they occur, even if no cash changes hands. This will mean a more accurate view of your business when the event occurs or transaction takes place. Especially in healthcare, the money for services can be delayed for a long period of time, and this may not give you a clear picture of your business if you did not count the activity until the bill is actually paid. A doctor's office visit in November may not be paid till June. In accrual counting, you would count this activity in January as opposed to June. This means that the accounting records events of income and expenses when the events occur, as opposed to when the cash is received. Alternatively, a company can use cash basis accounting which means that the revenue is recorded when the cash is received and expenses are recorded when the cash is spent.

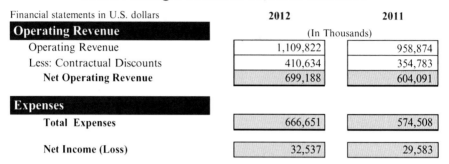

Fig. 5.2 Income section of Income Statement Expanded

In the revenue section of the income statement is a deduction for contractual discounts. Contractual discounts are discounts given to an insurance company for medical services established at your facility. These contractual discounts are negotiated with the insurance company when the hospital signs an agreement to provide care for the insurance company's clients. These contractual discounts can be a percentage of charge, a fee per service, or a lump-sum monthly payment for services. The revenue line would include the full charge for the procedures and services, and the contractual discounts will be presented as the expected deductions that relate to the contractual agreement. In Fig. 5.2, your revenue for the year was $1,109,822, and your accounting department decided that it is normal to collect 63 % of this figure, so the revenue would be reported as shown below with insurance contractual agreements of $410,634 and a net operating revenue of $699,565. After expenses of $666,651, your net income is $32,537. Remember that these contractual adjustments are early estimates and will be reconciled at the end of the year when the accounting books are closed for the year. These estimates must be fairly accurate or the hospital will have to be audited by an independent auditor.

Nonoperating Gains and Losses

Nonoperating gains and losses come from activities that occur outside of the business. Examples of these activities can be contributions or donations to the organization, gains and losses from investment activities, or gains and losses from property sales. These activities can be quite a significant part of the organization. At times, these gains and losses can make or break a company's financial status for their period.

The nonoperating revenue/expense section was added to Fig. 5.3 and shows an investment loss of $12,500 in 2011 and a gain of $15,000 in 2012. This could be from investments, bonds, or other investing activities. The second line is for

Buckeye Medical Center
Income Statement
Years Ending December 31, 2012 and 2011

Financial statements in U.S. dollars	2012	2011
Operating Revenue	(In Thousands)	
Operating Revenue	1,109,822	958,874
Less: Contractual Discounts	410,634	354,783
Net Operating Revenue	699,188	604,091
Operating Expenses		
Total Operating Expenses	633,565	524,684
Income From Operations	65,623	79,407
Non Operating Revenue (Expenses)		
Investment Income (loss)	15,000	(12,500)
Community Support and Charity	(55,682)	(45,893)
Other	7,596	8,569
Total Non Operating Income	(33,086)	(49,824)
Net Income (Loss)	32,537	29,583

Fig. 5.3 Non Operating Revenue section of Income Statement Expanded

community support or charity. The use of cash in this area represents free medical services provided to patients and also monies given to the community for medical and education programs such as a diabetic clinic or blood pressure screening and so forth. The "other" category represents revenues and expenses that are not related to the main operations of the business, such as parking lot fees, rental of space or equipment, or gift shop sales.

Expenses

The "expenses" line on the income statement refers to how the organization spends money for the operations of the business. In most general-purpose financial statements, healthcare costs are broken down into the following categories:

- Salaries and wages—nonphysicians
- Professional fees
- Employee benefits
- Supplies
- Purchased services

Buckeye Medical Center
Income Statement
Years Ending December 31, 2012 and 2011

Financial statements in U.S. dollars

	2012	2011
Operating Revenue	(In Thousands)	
Operating Revenue	1,109,822	958,874
Less: Contractual Discounts	410,634	354,783
Net Operating Revenue	699,188	604,091
Operating Expenses		
Salaries and Wages - Non Physician	221,504	181,562
Professional Fees	85,371	69,977
Employee Benefits	89,986	73,759
Supplies	69,220	56,738
Purchased Services	48,454	39,716
Facilities	29,995	24,586
Insurance	11,536	9,456
Utilities	9,229	7,565
Interest Expense	8,625	7,902
Depriciation and Amortization	41,532	34,042
Bad Debt	13,599	15,599
Other	4,514	3,782
Total Operating Expenses	633,565	524,684
Income From Operations	65,623	79,407
Non Operating Revenue (Expenses)		
Investment Income (loss0	15,000	(12,500)
Community Support and Charity	(55,682)	(45,893)
Other	7,596	8,569
Total Non Operating Income	(33,086)	(49,824)
Net Income (Loss)	32,537	29,583

Fig. 5.4 Expense section of Income Statement Expanded

- Facilities
- Insurance
- Utilities
- Interest expense
- Depreciation and amortization
- Bad debt
- Other

Most of these expenses can be easily understood. Figure 5.4 shows these expenses salaries, wages, and benefits are expenses tied to your employees.

"Professional fees" are for physician salaries. These can be broken down further into physician and professional staff (NP's, PA's, etc.), employee, and administrative expenses depending on the level of detail on the financial statements and the size of the organization. Supplies can be all included in one line or can be divided into medical supplies and drugs versus nonmedical supplies and drugs. "Purchased services" refers to services provided by outside vendors such as physics services, a mobile lithotripsy, or other billing services. "Administrative expenses" are expenses which are not directly tied to the medical business brought upon by managers, supervisors, and upper-level administrators. Rent, utilities, telephone, and IT expenses are all facility expenses which can be as detailed or combined on the financial statements as the organization wishes. Interest is expense does recognize for a current period.

Depreciation and amortization are two noncash accounts that represent the use of capital equipment, land, and buildings that are expressed as expenses over their useful lifetime. The hospital may buy a CT scanner that costs $700,000 and is expensed over a 7-year period which coincides with its useful life or how long this must be working at a high-quality level for the hospital. The depreciation expense every year for 7 years will be $100,000. This is not an actual cash distribution but recognition of the use of that asset. Bad debt is money for services that will never be collected for reasons such as the bankruptcy of a patient.

Importance of Income Statements

The income statement is one of the most important statements in a company's business. A business's ability to earn a consistent positive net income is a key decision driver for many external and internal decisions. It is used to look at the wealth of the organization to show whether the company is making or losing money. Creditors will use income statements to determine a company's ability to pay future and present debts. State and federal regulatory agencies and credentialing agencies will access a company's income statement to verify that that organization's financial status is adequate and viable. For management of the organization, this can be a detailed analysis of where revenue is coming into the organization and where money is being spent out of the organization. This review will help management decide how and where to make alterations in the company to improve the income statement.

It is important to remember that all financial statements will not look the same. The base format of "revenue minus expenses equals income" is a baseline standard. From there, each company will vary slightly as far as line items under each section. There is no standard format as far as how the line items are listed. Each company will create their financial statements as they see fit based on their business needs and industry requirements.

Further Reading

Cleverley W, Cleverley J, Song P. Essentials of health care finance. Sudbury, MA: Jones & Bartlett Learning; 2011.

Finkler S, Ward D. Accounting fundamentals for health care management. Sudbury, MA: Jones and Bartlett; 2006.

Gapenski L, Pink G. Understanding healthcare financial management. Chicago, IL: Health Administration Press; 2011.

Getzen T. Health economics and financing. Hoboken, NJ: Wiley; 2010.

Getzen T. Health economics and financing. Hoboken, NJ: Wiley; 2013.

Huss W, Coleman M. Start your own medical practice. Naperville, IL: Sphinx; 2006.

Keagy B, Thomas M. Essentials of physician practice management. San Francisco: Jossey-Bass; 2004.

Kongstvedt P. Managed care. Boston: Jones and Bartlett; 2004.

Marcinko D, Hetico H. The business of medical practice. New York: Springer; 2011.

Reiboldt J. Financial management of the medical practice. Chicago, IL: American Medical Association; 2011.

Solomon R. The physician manager's handbook. Sudbury, MA: Jones and Bartlett; 2008.

Yousem D, Beauchamp N. Radiology business practice. Philadelphia, PA: Saunders; 2008.

Chapter 6
Balance Sheet

Abstract The balance sheet is a financial statement which represents a record of the organizations' assets, liabilities, and net worth. The balance sheet can also be defined as the "statement of financial position," but the term "balance sheet" will be used in this book. This record always refers to a specific point in time. A balance sheet can be viewed at any point in time, but normally a business views this on a monthly basis and fiscal year basis. Assets are items that are worth money to you and are in your possession or are owed to you. Liabilities are debts that you owe for the assets. Net worth is the value of your company. The basic equation for the balance sheet is "assets equal liabilities plus net worth or shareholder's equity." It is called a balance sheet because both sides of the equation must be equal.

$$\text{Assets} = \text{Liabilities} + \text{Net Worth/Shareholders' Equity}$$

The balance sheet is used to take a look at your company in regard to assets and debts, as well as the ownership value.

The three parts of the balance sheet will have many different accounts within those sections. All of these details will differ based on the type of business. As with the income statement, there is not an exact template used for the balance sheet. The following balance sheet will showcase some general headings and sections. The balance sheet either can be laid out in a side-to-side manner with assets on one side and liabilities and net worth on the other or can be lined up vertically with the assets on top, the liabilities in the middle, and the net worth section on the bottom. A side-to-side manner will be utilized for this chapter.

Assets

Assets are items that you own in the company that have value to you. Some of these items can be in cash, in short-term interest-bearing items, or in receivables in which people owe you money. The asset section is broken down into current assets and

Fig. 6.1 Current asset
section of a balance sheet

ASSETS	
Current Assets	
Cash or Cash Equivalents	$57,561
Accounts receivable	212,568
(less allowances)	(78,650)
Inventory and Supplies	33,596
Temporary investment	17,953
Prepaid expenses	43,283
Total Current Assets	$286,311

long-term assets. Current assets are normally cash or something that will be redeemable for cash within a year. Figure 6.1 shows the current asset section of the balance sheet, with some subsets that normally appear under the current asset section.

Cash or Cash Equivalents—This section includes actual cash on hand or deposited at a local bank that is readily available. Other instruments considered cash are certified checks, money orders, savings accounts, and other temporary marketable securities. There are two requirements for items to be considered cash or cash equivalents. First, management must have intentions of converting the security into cash within 1 year or within the current operating cycle. Second, the security must be easily marketable and capable of being turned into cash fast. Currently the company has cash and cash equivalents of $57,561.

Accounts Receivable—Accounts receivable is the amount owed to you from your customers or patients. In a non-healthcare business, this would be recorded as sales on credit. In the healthcare business, this would be bills for patient services and medical supplies. The healthcare business is different in a sense that many of the bills will be sent to insurance companies rather than directly to the patients. This generally causes a delay in the receipt of these bills for services rendered. Also there are four major deductions or allowances for these patient bills.

Allowances

Contractual Allowances—This is the difference in the amount billed for patient service and the amount paid by the insurance company through a contractual agreement with the company. Because most major payers such as Medicare, Medicaid, and Blue Cross have a contractual relationship with your facility, payments are based on the terms of the contract and can sometimes be quite large.

Charity Allowances—This is an allowance for patients who are unable to pay for the care they require. It is the difference between the total of the charges in the actual payments from the patients. Charity allowances are normally based on the patient's income in relationship to the federal poverty levels.

Courtesy Allowances—These are special discounts for services rendered to special patients, such as employees, physicians, and clergy. These types of allowances have been decreasing over time due to increased rules and regulations from both government insurance programs and private pay insurance companies as well.

Allowance for Bad Debt—This is the amount of accounts receivable that will never be collected due to indigent patients, bankruptcy, deaths, and other reasons where the patients will never pay the bill.

The accounts receivable is $212,568 less the allowances of $78,650 for a net accounts receivable balance of $133,918.

Inventory and Supplies—This area of the balance sheet represents the items that are used in the delivery of healthcare. These can vary from patient care supplies such as needles, contrast for radiology exams, or replacement prosthesis. This category usually involves an allowance for any inventory supplies unexpectedly used in the hospital system within the next year or fiscal year. The inventory for this company shows a value of $33,596,000.

Temporary Investments—These are investments that will be redeemed for cash within the next year or fiscal period.

Prepaid Expenses—Prepaid expenses are payments received in advance for services to be used in the period of the next year. These can include rent, insurance payments, equipment leases, or other similar items. An example would be if you paid the lease cost for a portable lithotripsy unit in the hospital on a weekly basis. If you prepaid a lease by 6 months at $5,000 per month, then you would have a prepaid expense at a current asset of $30,000. A total amount of $43,283 is shown in prepaid expenses on the statement.

Fixed Assets

"Fixed assets" is the next major section of the asset division balance sheet. This section can also be known as long-term assets or plant, property, and equipment. The items in this category are expected to be kept by the organization for more than 1 year or a fiscal year. These are normally assets that produce revenues and can be used over and over again such as a building or medical equipment. The following listings under fixed assets are generally used, but each organization may have their own variation. Figure 6.2 shows the fixed asset section of the balance sheet.

Long-Term Investments—These are investments that cannot be redeemed for cash within the next year or fiscal period.

Land and Improvements—This section requires a historical or purchase price of land owned by the organization and any money spent to improve such land such as water and sewer lines, parking lots, or fences. Land held for investment purposes would not be shown in this section but would instead be shown in the investment section of the balance sheet. The company has 225,000 of land owned at this time.

Fig. 6.2 Fixed asset section
of a balance sheet

Fixed Assets	
Long-term investments	$145,693
Land	225,654
Buildings	357,623
(less accumulated depreciation)	(204,064)
Equipment	212,661
(less accumulated depreciation)	(102,596)
Furniture and fixtures	46,960
(less accumulated depreciation)	(25,663)
Other Assets (Intangibles)	53,014
Total Net Fixed Assets	**$709,282**

TOTAL ASSETS

Buildings Less Accumulated Depreciation—This area contains all the buildings owned by the company used in the normal course of business. These will contain the hospital building itself, hospital-owned physician offices, parking garages, and all other buildings to be used for operations. These items are listed at a value of their original costs less any depreciation on the income statement. The buildings for this company value at $357,623 and have claimed to depreciation of $204,064.

Equipment Less Accumulated Depreciation—All equipment owned by the company and used in operations is included in this section. This can include the MRI machine, surgical tables, hospital-owned ambulance, and all other equipment used in operations. This section can be broken down into three more categories: (1) fixed equipment, which is attached to the building in which it is located such as an elevator or generator; (2) major movable equipment such as automobiles or a portable x-ray device; and (3) minor equipment associated with a short useful life span such as patient gowns or wastebaskets. These are listed on the balance sheet at their purchase price less any depreciation claimed by the company. Buckeye Medical Center currently ends $212,661 in equipment, and they have claimed $102,596 against equipment.

Furniture and Fixtures Less Accumulated Depreciation—This item can be used on a balance sheet to include office furniture, storage bins, counters, and other items of similar nature to be used in operations. These are listed on the balance sheet at their purchase price less any depreciation claimed by the company. Furniture and fixtures for this company are valued at $46,960 less accumulated depreciation of $25,663.

Other Expenses—This is an area that includes assets that are intangible such as patents, royalty arrangements, and copyrights. These are assets that have a value placed on them which is estimated by the company in regard to how much future revenue the company will receive from them. Goodwill typically reflects the value of intangible assets such as a strong brand name, employee and customer relations, and any proprietary technology. Other assets are valued at $53,014.

LIABILITIES

Current Liabilities	
Accounts payable	$62,975
Short-term notes	26,397
Current portion of long-term notes	56,396
Interest payable	2,569
Accrued payroll	7,852
Other Accrued Expenses	86,319
Total Current Liabilities	**$242,508**
Long-term Liabilities	
Mortgage	$175,963
Other long-term liabilities	167,182
Total Long-Term Liabilities	**$343,145**

Fig. 6.3 Current liability section of a balance sheet

Liabilities

Liabilities are amounts owed to vendors, employees, and other organizations. These are basically the claims of creditors against assets of the business. There are two types of liabilities: short-term liabilities or obligations that must be paid within the next year or fiscal cycle of the company and long-term liabilities which are obligations that will be paid back over a longer period of time in the next year or fiscal period. Figure 6.3 shows the liability section of the balance sheet.

Current Liabilities

This section includes accounts payable, notes payable, taxes payable, and accrued expenses payable over the next year. Specific sections are shown in the below paragraph:

Accounts payable—This is the amount that you owe suppliers or other creditors for goods and services that you have purchased but have not yet paid for. For example, this can be in the form of a bill for surgical supplies that were used in a case but for which payment has not been made. The accounts payable shows that this company does vendor the amount of $62,975.

Short-term notes payable—This is normally the amount you owe to banks or other lending institutions for a loan or line of credit that is due within the next 12 months. Short-term notes outstanding for Buckeye medical center is $26,397.

Current portion of long-term debt—Some of the monies due in the next year for long-term debt are presented in this section. The current portion of long-term debt owed by Buckeye is $56,396.

Accrued payroll—This is money which is owed to employees for hours worked. Most institutions pay their employees a week or two after their actually work their hours. The amount owed for that time is the accrued payroll. The employees are due $7,852 from this company at this point in time.

Interest payable—This represents any monies due for interest on any credit items. Interest is owed by this company in the amount of $2,569.

Taxes payable—Any taxes that are to be paid in the next year including payroll, business, and other related taxes to the state, federal, or local governments.

Other current liabilities—the current liability section can be broken down into many more current assets which have similar obligations as those listed above. These can include insurance payable, rent payable, lease expense payable, legal fees payable, etc.; other current liabilities for this company amount to $86,319.

Long-Term Liabilities

Long-term liability sections are any debts that must be paid by your company more than a year from now. Some of these liabilities include bank loans, notes payable to shareholders or stockholders, long-term obligations to other companies, or other long-term debt. Mortgages and others are listed in this balance sheet, but this section can include a multitude of line items depending on the company. The long-term liabilities for this company are $175,963 for mortgage loans and $167,182 for other long-term liabilities.

Net Assets or Shareholders Equity

This represents a difference of assets minus liabilities. This will be viewed differently in regard to whether the company is for profit or not for profit. The asset and liability sections are pretty similar in both situations. The difference occurs in the equity section, which can include either shareholder equity or net assets.

For-Profit Companies—The for-profit company is owned by shareholders and distributes money among the owners. In this type of company, the difference between the assets and liabilities is representative of the owners' interest or worth to the stockholders. The section can be referred to as owners' equity or shareholders' equity.

Common and/or Preferred Stock—This is the owners' interest in a company with regard to the stock that they own. Some companies list common and preferred depending on their structure type. The calculation for this section is assets minus liabilities minus retained earnings minus any other items in the shareholders' equity section equals value of stock in the company. Common stock for this company is $184,873 and $98,693 for preferred stock.

For Profit		Not For Profit	
Shareholders' Equity		**Net Assets**	
Capital stock	$184,873	Unrestricted Funds	$184,873
Preferred Stock	$98,693	Temporarily Restricted Funds	$98,693
Retained earnings	126,374	Permanently Restricted Funds	$126,374
Total Shareholders' Equity	$409,940	**Total Net Assets**	$409,940
TOTAL LIABILITIES & EQUITY	$995,593	**TOTAL LIABILITIES & EQUITY**	$995,593

Fig. 6.4 Shareholders' equity section of a for-profit company and a net asset section of a not-for-profit company

Retained Earnings—Retained earnings are the amount of profit earned by the company which was reinvested into the business as opposed to paid out to shareholders or spent on acquisitions. If the company had $1 million in existing retained earnings and earned a profit of $500,000 in the same year which was also invested into the company, then the new retained earnings figure would be $1.5 million. The retained earnings held by this company amount to $226,374.

Not-for-Profit Companies—The balance sheet changes for nonprofit companies because there are no actual owners of the company. Since there are no actual owners of the company, the difference between assets and liabilities is shown as assets or holdings as opposed to equity to a stockholder. Instead, nonprofits would use the same equation of assets minus liabilities equals net assets, but the net assets would be broken down into unrestricted, temporarily restricted, and permanently restricted assets.

Unrestricted Funds—These funds can be used for any purpose which the company sees fit for the betterment of the organization. Unrestricted funds for this company are $184,873.

Temporarily Restricted Funds—These funds are normally restricted for a period of time, until certain events occur, or reserved for specific purposes. These amount to $98,693.

Permanently Restricted Funds—Considered permanently restricted, these funds can only be used for a specific purpose and restrictions can never be removed. This can be the case when a donor contributes money to an organization and they give specific directions and specifications of how that money will be used for the organization. The permanently restricted funds for Buckeye medical center are $126,374.

Figure 6.4 shows the two variations for the equity section of the balance sheet, and Figs. 6.5 and 6.6 show the complete balance sheets for both for-profit and not-for-profit companies. You will notice that the total assets and total liabilities & equity are equal to each other. That is, the basis of the balance sheet is that the asset & liabilities columns must be equal or balance.

Buckeye Medical Center

Balance Sheet - For-Profit

31-Dec-12
(all numbers in $000)

ASSETS		LIABILITIES	
Current Assets		**Current Liabilities**	
Cash or Cash Equivalents	$57,561	Accounts payable	$62,975
Accounts receivable	212,568	Short-term notes	26,397
(less allowances)	(78,650)	Current portion of long-term notes	56,396
Inventory and Supplies	33,596	Interest payable	2,569
Temporary investment	17,953	Accrued payroll	7,852
Prepaid expenses	43,283	Other Accrued Expenses	86,319
Total Current Assets	**$286,311**	**Total Current Liabilities**	**$242,508**
Fixed Assets		**Long-term Liabilities**	
Long-term investments	$145,693	Mortgage	$175,963
Land	225,654	Other long-term liabilities	167,182
Buildings	357,623	**Total Long-Term Liabilities**	**$343,145**
(less accumulated depreciation)	(204,064)		
Equipment	212,661		
(less accumulated depreciation)	(102,596)	**Shareholders' Equity**	
Furniture and fixtures	46,960	Capital stock	$184,873
(less accumulated depreciation)	(25,663)	Preferred Stock	$98,693
Other Assets (Intangibles)	53,014	Retained earnings	$126,374
Total Net Fixed Assets	**$709,282**	**Total Shareholders' Equity**	**$409,940**
TOTAL ASSETS	**$995,593**	**TOTAL LIABILITIES & EQUITY**	**$995,593**

Fig. 6.5 Complete balance sheet for a for-profit company

Buckeye Medical Center

Balance Sheet - Not-For-Profit

31-Dec-12
(all numbers in $000)

ASSETS		LIABILITIES	
Current Assets		**Current Liabilities**	
Cash or Cash Equivalents	$57,561	Accounts payable	$62,975
Accounts receivable	212,568	Short-term notes	26,397
(less allowances)	(78,650)	Current portion of long-term notes	56,396
Inventory and Supplies	33,596	Interest payable	2,569
Temporary investment	17,953	Taxes payable	7,852
Prepaid expenses	43,283	Accrued payroll	86,319
Total Current Assets	**$286,311**	**Total Current Liabilities**	**$242,508**
Fixed Assets		**Long-term Liabilities**	
Long-term investments	$145,693	Mortgage	$175,963
Land	225,654	Other long-term liabilities	167,182
Buildings	357,623	**Total Long-Term Liabilities**	**$343,145**
(less accumulated depreciation)	(204,064)		
Equipment	212,661		
(less accumulated depreciation)	(102,596)	**Net Assets**	
Furniture and fixtures	46,960	Unrestricted Funds	$184,873
(less accumulated depreciation)	(25,663)	Temporarily Restricted Funds	$98,693
Other Assets (Intangibles)	53,014	Permanently Restricted Funds	$126,374
Total Net Fixed Assets	**$709,282**	**Total Net Assets**	**$409,940**
TOTAL ASSETS	**$995,593**	**TOTAL LIABILITIES & EQUITY**	**$995,593**

Fig. 6.6 Complete balance sheet for a not-for-profit company

Further Reading

Cleverley W, Cleverley J, Song P. Essentials of health care finance. Sudbury, MA: Jones & Bartlett Learning; 2011.

Finkler S, Ward D. Accounting fundamentals for health care management. Sudbury, MA: Jones and Bartlett; 2006.

Gapenski L, Pink G. Understanding healthcare financial management. Chicago, IL: Health Administration Press; 2011.

Getzen T. Health economics and financing. Hoboken, NJ: Wiley; 2010.

Getzen T. Health economics and financing. Hoboken, NJ: Wiley; 2013.

Huss W, Coleman M. Start your own medical practice. Naperville, IL: Sphinx; 2006.

Keagy B, Thomas M. Essentials of physician practice management. San Francisco, CA: Jossey-Bass; 2004.

Kongstvedt P. Managed care. Boston, MA: Jones and Bartlett; 2004.

Marcinko D, Hetico H. The business of medical practice. New York: Springer; 2011.

Reiboldt J. Financial management of the medical practice. Chicago, IL: American Medical Association; 2011.

Solomon R. The physician manager's handbook. Sudbury, MA: Jones and Bartlett; 2008.

Yousem D, Beauchamp N. Radiology business practice. Philadelphia, PA: Saunders; 2008.

Chapter 7
Statement of Cash Flows

Abstract The statement of cash flows is the third required financial statement for all companies. The cash flow statement is a complement to the income statement in the balance sheet. It was added as a requirement with the income statement and the balance sheet in 1988 as required financial documents for all businesses by the US Security and Exchange Commission. The statement shows the change of actual cash flow in a company over a period of time. As we described earlier, some expenses and incomes do not actually represent real cash dollars. This document describes the actual cash flow into and out of the entity. It starts with cash at the beginning of a period such as a year or physical period and then adds and subtracts the actual cash flow during the period. The income statement presented earlier is concerned about the company making a profit. Statement of cash flows is concerned about the company generating enough cash to be viable and sustainable. The company generates a surplus of cash; then the organization can be considered viably stable if they generate more cash than they spend. In general there are three sections or activities in the statement of cash flows: *operating activities, investing activities, and financing activities*. People and groups who are mainly interested in the cash flow statements are accounting personnel, lenders and creditors, shareholders, employees and contractors, and potential investors into the business.

About This Statement

This statement can be described as the most complicated but can be the most important one since it actually shows how much cash a business has. Most positions and administrators never really have to worry about figuring this report out. This is normally done by accounting software programs in the accountants of the organization. What is important for physicians and administrators is that we have an understanding of where the numbers for this statement come from and basically how this report is generated. This chapter will review the two different types of statement of cash flows and give a basic understanding of how these reports are generated and reviewed. A couple sample statements of cash flow will be presented.

Typical Cash Flow Statement

The cash flow statement explains how changes occurred in a certain period of cash and cash equivalents. Cash includes currency, cash on hand, and demand deposits. Cash equivalents can be in the form of very liquid investments that can be readily turned into currency. A sample statement of cash flows is shown in Fig. 7.1 and each section is explained below.

This fictitious company had a net income on the income statement of $600. The first thing we must do is add in depreciation and amortization since these are non-cash items. Next you account for the changes in current assets and liabilities. It can also be seen that the building was purchased for $350 using cash and money was paid upon the principle of a mortgage loan which also was paid in cash. In this year, the increase in cash for the company was $220 which is added to the beginning cash value of $300 for an end of your cash number of $520.

ACME
Statement Of Cash Flows
Years Ending December 31, 2012

	2012
Cash Flows from Operating Activities	
Net Income	$600
Additions (Sources of Cash)	
Depreciation or Amortization	140
Increase in Accounts Payable	60
Increase in Accrued Payroll	15
Subtractions	
Increase in Accounts Receivable	−165
Increase in Inventory	−30
Cash Flows from Investing Activities	
Purchase of Building	−350
Cash Flows from Financing Activities	
Payment of Mortgage Principal	−$50
NET INCREASE/(DECREASE) IN CASH	$220
CASH, BEGINNING OF YEAR	300
CASH, END OF YEAR	$520

Fig. 7.1   Typical cash flow statement

Statement of Cash Flows Activities

There are three sections of the statement of cash flows which include *operating activities, investing activities, and financing activities.*

Operating Activities

Operating activities include any production, sales, and delivery of the product or service for the company. Examples of operating activities are office visits, surgeries, lab procedures, etc. Operating activities normally generate cash and the related expenses normally spend cash. There are some activities that do not consume or spend cash. This statement will convert the items reported on the income statement from the accrual basis of accounting to the cash basis of accounting. These are the expenses in revenues that must be added and subtracted in the statement of cash flows.

Investing Activities

Investing activities are any transactions that involve purchasing shares or ownership units in another company, stock, bond, or other outside company ownerships. These activities that show and increase or decrease in investments in assets of the company. Types of activity included investing our increases or decreases in marketable securities, sale or purchase of buildings and land, and purchases of equipment.

Financing Activities

Items shown in this area include increases or decreases in mortgages, transfers of cash to parent or subsidiary organizations, changes in equity sections of the organization, and other changes in long-term debt.

Increases and Decreases in Cash Flow

There are many changes of cash flow related to activities of the company. Some of these activities will increase cash, while others will decrease the cash in the business. Figure 7.2 displays some of these increases and decreases of cash flow.

This can be further detailed for changes in the balance sheet. Figure 7.3 shows some changes in cash relating to balance sheet account changes.

Cash Inflows or Sources of Cash		
Operating Activities	**Investing Activities**	**Financing Activities**
Cash received from customers	Collections from loans and financing activities	Issuing long-term debt
Interest income	Selling of debt instruments	Issuing equity securities
Dividends income	Sale of equity instruments	
Other operating receipts and cash	Sale of useful assets	
Cash Outflows or Uses of Cas h		
Operating Activities	**Investing Activities**	**Financing Activities**
Payments to suppliers	Purchase of useful assets	Dividend payments
Payments to employees	Purchase of debt instruments	Acquiring your own securities back
Payments on interest	Purchasing equity instruments	Repayment of borrowings
Payments for income taxes	Addition of a loan	
Other operating cash payments		

Fig. 7.2   Activities that increase and decrease cash flow

Inflows Of Cash	Outflows Of Cash
A decrease in an asset account	An increase in an asset account
An increase in the liability count	A decrease in the liability count
An increase in an equity account	A decrease in an equity account

Fig. 7.3   Changes in cash related to balance sheet changes

In summary, if an asset account increases, then the result is a decrease in cash. If the asset account increases, then this results in an increase in cash. In liabilities and equity, an increase in either one will mirror an increase in cash. Likewise a decrease in either one will result in a decrease in cash.

Direct Versus Indirect Statements of Cash Flow

There are two different types of statements of cash flow. They are the direct method and indirect method? The direct method starts with the beginning cash balance and shows direct increases and decreases of cash in different areas. The direct method is one where you go through the three sections of the cash flow statement and in you show how much cash was directly spent on each section of the statement. If you received $100,000 customers, then you would see cash increases of $100,000 in that section. This will become clearer as you review the different types of statements of cash flow. The indirect method is a variation of the direct method. It makes adjustments to account for noncash items that are included in the balance sheet and income statement such as depreciation. Noncash items are added and subtracted in this method. In the indirect type of statement of cash flows, one would see conditions and subtractions for noncash items in the different sections. For example, depreciation of $100,000 in the expense section of the income statement would be shown as $100,000 addition in the cash flow statement. Whichever method is used by the corporation, the end product for the final calculation figure will be exactly the same. More firms utilize the indirect method of statement of cash flows because it gives a more accurate statement when using accrual-based accounting.

Direct Statement of Cash Flow

Figure 7.4 shows operating activities and related clash cash flow changes under the direct method. This is for a fictitious company and not representative of another company in this book. You will notice in this statement that the sources and uses of cash are directly shown. $10,500 was received from payments in cash, for example, and interest amount of $8,000 was paid directly in cash as well. The rest of the statement closes exactly in this respect as we move through the rest of the accounts for a bottom-line change in cash flow.

Indirect Statement of Cash Flow

The indirect method of cash flow statement is reported by adjusting net income for revenues, expenses, gains, and losses that appear on the income statement that do not affect cash. Figure 7.5 below reviews how changes in different accounts affect the increase or decrease in cash.

Figure 7.6 shows an example of what an indirect statement of cash flow would look like.

Cash Flows From Operating Activities Under The Direct Method	
Cash collections from sales or services	Sales less increases in Accounts Receivable minus bad debt OR Sales plus decreases in Accounts Receivable minus bad debt
Cash payments to suppliers or vendors	Cost of goods sold plus increases in inventory OR less decreases in inventory AND minus increases in accounts payable or plus decreases in accounts payable
Other income/expense	Plus or minus other income/expenses
Payments for interest	Interest expense cash value
Dividends/withdrawals	Dividend/withdrawals paid plus increase in dividends payable OR minus decreases in dividends payable
Cash paid for taxes	Texas expense minus increase in accrued taxes payable OR plus decreases in accrued taxes payable AND decreases and prepaid tax OR increases in prepaid tax

Fig. 7.4 How operating activities affect cash flow under the direct method of a cash flow statement

Cash Flows from Investing Activities

The formula for figuring out the cash flows from investing activities utilizes the following equation:

\+ Proceeds from sale of assets
− Purchases of property and equipment
= Total net cash provided (used) by investing activities

Cash Flows from Financing Activities

The formula for figuring out the cash flows from financing activities utilizes the following equation:

\+ Net borrowing under line of credit agreement
+ Proceeds from new borrowings

Adjustments to reconcile net income to net cash provided by operating activities under the Indirect method.	
Depreciation	Add to Net Income to Reconcile
Amortization of Bond Premium	Deduct from net Income to Reconcile
Amortization of Bond Discount	Add to Net Income to Reconcile
Gain on Sale of Equipment	Deduct from net Income to Reconcile
Loss on Sale of Equipment	Add to Net Income to Reconcile
Decrease in Accounts Receivable	Add to Net Income to Reconcile
Increase in Accounts Receivable	Deduct from net Income to Reconcile
Decrease in Inventory	Add to Net Income to Reconcile
Increase in Inventory	Deduct from net Income to Reconcile
Decrease in Accounts Payable	Deduct from net Income to Reconcile
Increase in Accounts Payable	Add to Net Income to Reconcile
Decrease in Accrued Expenses	Deduct from net Income to Reconcile
Increase in Accrued Expenses	Add to Net Income to Reconcile
Decrease in Prepaid Expenses	Add to Net Income to Reconcile
Increase in Prepaid Expenses	Deduct from net Income to Reconcile
Decrease in Taxes Payable	Deduct from net Income to Reconcile
Increase in Taxes Payable	Increase in Cash Flow

Fig. 7.5 How operating activities affect cash flow under the direct method of a cash flow statement

− Repayment of loans
− Principal payments under capital lease obligations
− Dividends/distributions/withdrawals paid
+ Proceeds from issuance of stock
+ Partner/owner capital contributions
= Total net cash provided (used) by financing activities

   The section should now be added together to see the cash provided from operations, investing, and financing at the time of the cash flow statement. At this point, one can analyze the cash flow statement for the positives and negatives of the company. Figure 7.7 shows an example of what an indirect statement of cash flow would look like. This indirect statement works in a different direction than the direct statement. It starts with the net income from the income statement. It then adds

Statement of Cash Flows - Direct Method Sample

Cash flows from (used in) operating activities

Period ending	31-Dec-12	
Cash receipts from customers	10,500	
Cash paid to suppliers and employees	−2,500	
Cash generated from operations (**sum**)	**8,000**	
Interest paid	−4,000	
Income taxes paid	−3,000	
Net cash flows from operating activities		**1,000**

Cash flows from (used in) investing activities

Proceeds from the sale of equipment	8,500	
Dividends received	5,000	
Net cash flows from investing activities		**13500**

Cash flows from (used in) financing activities

Dividends paid	−3,500	
Net cash flows used in financing activities		**−3,500**
Net increase in cash and cash equivalents		**11,000**
Cash and cash equivalents, beginning of year		**2,000**
Cash and cash equivalents, end of year		**13000**

Fig. 7.6 Typical cash flow statement using the direct method

Statement of Cash Flows - Indirect Method Sample

Period ending	*12/31/2012*
Net income	**35,126**

Operating activities, cash flows provided by or used in:

Depreciation and amortization	3,500
Adjustments to net income	2,500
Decrease (increase) in accounts receivable	20,115
Increase (decrease) in liabilities (A/P, taxes payable)	125,685
Decrease (increase) in inventories	0
Increase (decrease) in other operating activities	−160,000
Net cash flow from operating activities	26,926

Investing activities, cash flows provided by or used in:

Capital expenditures	−12,005
Investments	−150,000
Other cash flows from investing activities	2,500
Net cash flows from investing activities	−159,505

Financing activities, cash flows provided by or used in:

Dividends paid	−25,968
Sale (repurchase) of stock	−10,255
Increase (decrease) in debt	101,122
Other cash flows from financing activities	120,461
Net cash flows from financing activities	185,360
Net increase (decrease) in cash and cash equivalents	52,781

Fig. 7.7 Typical cash flow statement using the indirect method

noncash items such as depreciation and then adds or subtracts, respectively, for increases and decreases in each account of the balance sheet statement. Although this example of the direct cash flow statement sample is mathematically different, in the end, these will both end up at the same amount at the bottom line.

Further Reading

Cleverley W, Cleverley J, Song P. Essentials of health care finance. Sudbury, MA: Jones & Bartlett Learning; 2011.

Finkler S, Ward D. Accounting fundamentals for health care management. Sudbury, MA: Jones and Bartlett; 2006.

Gapenski L, Pink G. Understanding healthcare financial management. Chicago: Health Administration Press; 2011.

Getzen T. Health economics and financing. Hoboken, NJ: Wiley; 2010.

Getzen T. Health economics and financing. Hoboken: Wiley; 2013.

Huss W, Coleman M. Start your own medical practice. Naperville, IL: Sphinx; 2006.

Keagy B, Thomas M. Essentials of physician practice management. San Francisco: Jossey-Bass; 2004.

Kongstvedt P. Managed care. Boston: Jones and Bartlett; 2004.

Marcinko D, Hetico H. The business of medical practice. New York: Springer; 2011.

Reiboldt J. Financial management of the medical practice. Chicago, IL: American Medical Association; 2011.

Solomon R. The physician manager's handbook. Sudbury, MA: Jones and Bartlett; 2008.

Yousem D, Beauchamp N. Radiology business practice. Philadelphia, PA: Saunders; 2008.

Chapter 8
Financial Ratios

Abstract Financial ratios are a way of analyzing your business's financial health. The income statement and balance sheet are used to create ratios and statistics in order to evaluate how your company is performing financially. These ratios can be used to compare against your previous periods, against other businesses within your business sector, or against benchmarks provided by organizations and companies. Being in the medical business, you're already using ratios in your practice of some sort. The purpose of financial ratios is to assist you with information in decision-making in your practice in the form of ratios and comparisons. There are four main types of ratios that we will examine: profitability ratios, liquidity ratios, debt ratios, and asset ratios, along with some additional ratios that hospitals use. Each of these four types of ratios contains numerous possible ratios. Although the scope of this text is not to cover every possible ratio in existence, the purpose is to give you a brief description, a formula, and an example of financial ratios that are most popular in healthcare business. Some of the ratios included are total profit margin, days in accounts receivable, days cash on hand, and return on equity, just to name a few. The following will display the most important ratios that are utilized in healthcare, and sample calculations will be provided by the income statement and balance sheet of Buckeye Medical Center from Chaps. 5 and 6.

Profitability Ratios

Profitability ratios are ways in which a firm looks at its profits as compared to its sales, assets, and ownership in the company. It is able to see whether it is making a good profit in comparison to these other financial numbers. These are the major ratios viewed by banks, lenders, and investors for analysis purposes.

Total Margin or Profit Margin

Definition/Purpose: The profit margin ratio is one of the most popular ratios that businesses review. It looks at the company's net income or bottom line and compares it to the operating income. The higher the margins of the total margin, the higher the company's ability to make money.

Formula: total or profit margin = net income/total operating revenue
Total margin = 32,537/699,188 = 0.046 or 4.6 %

Rational and Standards: The profit margin is 4.6 % which means that the hospital will make 4.6 cents on each dollar of revenue that it earns. The industry average for this margin is 5 %. The average in our example is a little low as compared to the industry average.

Operating Margin

Definition/Purpose: The operating margin is similar to the profit margin but is a measure of the operating income compared to operating revenues. This is the most used financial ratios by hospitals in regard to profitability.

Formula: operating margin = operating income/operating revenues
Operating margin = 65,623/699,188 = 0.093 or 9.3 %

Rational and Standards: This ratio shows that the company is making 9.3 cents on every dollar of revenue earned. This is higher than the total margin of 4.6 %. This means that the company makes most of its money from their main core of business as opposed to investments in other nonoperating activities. The industry average of 3.1 % in our example is high above the average.

Return on Assets (ROA)

Definition/Purpose: This ratio shows how much profit is generated from every dollar spent on the assets of the company. It basically tells a company how they are using their assets to generate revenue for the business. The higher the ratio, the more the business uses assets for their business purpose.

Formula: return on assets = net income/total assets
Return on assets = 32,537/995,893 = 0.0032 or 3.2 %

Rational and Standards: Buckeye Medical Center's return on assets is not very high. The industry standard is 4.8 %. This would mean that Buckeye has too many assets in their portfolio and probably thinks about selling off some land or buildings and other unused assets in order to improve this ratio.

Return on Equity (ROE)

Definition/Purpose: The return on equity is similar to the return on assets, but the net income is ratios against the total equity of the company. This ratio shows how well the company is able to generate for every dollar invested in equity. This equation is used in for-profit companies. A very similar equation will be displayed next.

Formula: return on equity = net income/total equity
Return on equity = 32,537/409,940 = 0.079 or 79 %

Rational and Standards: The industry standard for healthcare is 8.4 %, and we can see from this equation that our company is a little below the standard. This figure can be improved by buying back some of its stock or spending or distributing some of its retained earnings.

Return on Funds

Definition/Purpose: This formula is exactly the same as the return on equity described earlier except that this is used for not-for-profit companies. The only difference is that we replace the words total equity with total funds.

Formula: return on funds = net income/total funds
Return on equity = 32,537/409,940 = 0.079 or 79 %

Rational and Standards: The industry standard for healthcare is 8.4 %, and we can see from this equation that our company is a little below the standard. This figure can be improved by spending some of its funds.

Liquidity Ratios

Liquidity ratios are ways in which the firm can easily view the firm's financial status to see if it can meet financial obligations in the short term and also see if these funds show opportunities for growth, investment, or other ways to earn a profit. These ratios went through the following two questions: Is this firm able to meet its obligations in the near future, and how much availability of funds is there to find other ways to make profits?

Current Ratio

Definition/Purpose: This ratio compares the firm's current assets with the current liabilities. This is the simplest calculation to make sure that the firm can pay for its short-term obligations with the cash and cash equivalents in hand and in the bank.

Formula: current ratio=current assets/current liabilities
Current ratio=286,311/24,258=1.18

Rational and Standards: This is an unhealthy number in the current ratio. This means that the firm can provide $1.18 for every one dollar of current liabilities that the firm owes.

Days in Accounts Receivable, Average Collection Period, and Days Sales Outstanding

Definition/Purpose: The accounts receivable measures the effectiveness of the firm collecting payments for services rendered. It represents the average number of days it takes to collect for services that was rendered. This is very relevant in medicine since most of the billings are through insurance companies and government providers. It is important to manage the amount of time that the average receivables are paid.

Formula: days in accounts receivable=*net patient accounts receivable*/(net patient service revenue/365)
Days in accounts receivable=133,918/(699,188/365)=69.93 days

Rational and Standards: For the Buckeye Medical Center, it takes approximately 69.9 days from the time a patient is billed for services until the cash is received in the company. The average in the industry is 73 days. Most companies like to see this numbers less than 40–50 days as a standard of practice in their institution. The higher the Medicaid and Medicare services are in your company, the more challenging it is to meet this market.

Days Cash on Hand

Definition/Purpose: This is a very important ratio for any business. It implies how many days of expenses that the current firm can pay with cash on hand today. In other words, if for some reason no cash is paid for services for a time period, how long could the company be able to pay bills with its current cash on hand?

Formula: days cash on hand=*cash*+*marketable securities*/ (expenses−depreciation−provision for uncollectibles)/365
Days cash on hand = 57,561/(633,565−41,532−13,559)/365=36.3 days

Rational and Standards: This firm's days cash on hand are 36.3 days. This is slightly higher than the industry average of 34.6. If no payments were received after today, then this firm would only be able to last 36 days with his current cash on hand to pay bills. There was an incident back in 2008 where the CMS stopped making payments for Medicaid and Medicare bills. This will be a very relevant ratio for situations like this.

Quick Ratio

Definition/Purpose: The quick ratio is also known as the "acid test." This ratio looks at your most liquid assets in comparison to your current liabilities. This test lets you know whether or not the business can meet obligations even in adverse conditions.

Formula: quick ratio = (total current assets − total inventory)/total current liabilities
Quick ratio = (286,311 − 33,596)/242,508 = 1.04

Rational and Standards: While this ratio is more relevant to other businesses that have high amounts of inventory for sales, the best figures are between 0.5 and 1. In medicine, this ratio is not that relevant unless your business is in the sales of medical supplies, DME, or other types of sales have inventory.

Return on Assets Ratio

Definition/Purpose: This ratio is a relationship between the profits of your company and your total assets. It shows how effective your company's assets are utilized in order to make a profit.

Formula: return on assets = profit before taxes/total assets
Return on assets = 32,537/995,593 = 0.032 or 32 %

Rational and Standards: This means that 3.2 cents profit is generated for each dollar and assets of the company. This is numbered; it needs to be compared with historical performance and peer hospitals in the industry.

Debt Ratios

Debt ratios are ways to measure how stable the firm is in its ability to pay off long-term debts. While these are important to the members of the company, banks, creditors, or lending institutions like to examine these ratios.

Debt Ratio

Definition/Purpose: The debt ratio measures the amount of assets owned by the firm that are obligated in the form of debt. In other words, what is the percentage of your assets that are financed by some kind of creditor or lending institution.

Formula: debt ratio = total debt/total assets
Debt ratio = 343,145/995,593 = 0.34 or 34 %

Rational and Standards: This shows that the firm has 34 % of its assets funded by some sort of debt. This is a pretty good value for this company since the industry average is 42.3 %.

Debt to Equity Ratio

Definition/Purpose: The debt ratio and a debt to equity ratio provide much of the same information with a slight variation. This ratio tells us that the creditors have supplied a certain percentage for each dollar of equity capital.

Formula: debt to equity ratio = total debt/total equity
Debt to equity ratio = 343,145,409,940 = 0.83

Rational and Standards: The industry average is 73.3 % and this firm is over that percentage by 10 points. This means the creditors contribute $0.83 on each dollar of equity capital. This firm may need to reduce this number.

Equity Financing Ratio

Definition/Purpose: This ratio measures the strength of the equity in the business as compared to total assets of business. The closer this number is to 1, the better the number is.

Formula: equity financing ratio = fund balance or equity balance/total assets
Equity financing ratio = 409,940/995,593 = 0.41

Rational and Standards: This equation tells us that 41 % of the businesses assets are owned by the company's equity.

Working Capital

Definition/Purpose: Working capital is the current assets less your current liabilities which shows you how much cash you have on hand.

Formula: working capital = total current assets − total current liabilities
Working capital = 286,311 − 242,508 = 43,803

Rational & Standards: Buckeye Medical Center has available $43,803 in working capital; since this number is positive, then they enough is cash to pay an current blus plus an excess.

Asset Management Ratios

Asset management ratios or activity ratios are designed to determine how effectively the firm's assets are managed. These ratios ask a question of whether or not the type and amount of assets on company balance sheet reasonable or not, especially in the eyes of lending institutions when authorities to borrow money to buy to expand.

Fixed Asset Turnover Cash Ratio or Fixed Asset Utilization Ratio

Definition/Purpose: This ratio measures the utilization of plant equipment. This will show how much revenue of each one dollar of fixed assets generates.

Formula: fixed asset turnover = total revenues/net fixed assets
Fixed asset turnover = 699,188,709,282 = 0.98

Rational and Standards: This ratio indicates that $0.98 revenue is produced for each one dollar of fixed assets. This is a relatively new low number for the industry as the average is 2.2. This firm may not be utilizing its fixed assets as productively as other comparative companies.

Other Ratios

This last group of ratios are ones mostly used by hospitals. These can be important indicators of financial well-being. These ratios measure how many days a patient is in a hospital, how many beds are filled, or how much an average patient charge is. These can also be called operating indicator ratios.

Net Price per Discharge

Definition/Purpose: This measures the average revenue collected for each patient on discharge.

Formula: net price per discharge = net inpatient revenue/total discharges

Rational and Standards: The industry standard is by $5,210 per discharge.

Outpatient Revenue Percentage

Definition/Purpose: This looks at the mix between outpatients and inpatients. We look to see what percentage of outpatients is compared to inpatients in the hospital setting.

Formula: outpatient revenue percentage = net outpatient revenue/net patient service
    revenue

Rational and Standards: Companies like to keep an eye on their percentage of outpatients. Outpatients are more profitable than inpatients. They also like to keep their
outpatient rate as high as possible.

Occupancy Percentage

Definition/Purpose: This is a measurement of how the hospital beds are utilized by
patients. Patient beds are assets and hospitals should make sure that they are being
utilized.

Formula: outpatient revenue percentage = net outpatient revenue/net patient service
    revenue

Rational and Standards: The industry average is 34.5 %. Obviously the higher occu-
pancy rate, the better it is financially for the hospital.

Average Length of Stay (ALOS)

Definition/Purpose: This is a basic measurement of how long an average patient
stays in a hospital.

Formula: ALOS=inpatient days/total discharges

Rational and Standards: The average in the industry is 5.1 days. Our example here
has a longer length of stay. When examining this we need to also look at the case-
mix index of the patients. Some patients may have more complicated medical conditions and require longer stays in some facilities than others.

Cost per Discharge

Definition/Purpose: This is the measurement of the average cost per discharge for
each patient. This gives us an idea of how much revenue to expect when an individual becomes an in patient at the hospital. The industry standard is $5,246.

Formula: discharge = inpatient operating expenses/total discharges

Rational and Standards: The industry average is $5,246 per patient. Once again, you
need to review your case mix for these patients relative to other hospitals on the
industry average.

Benchmarking

Benchmarking is a process of reviewing one business's results against another business's results for comparison and analysis. It is the process of comparing performance results of separate and sometimes competing organizations in order to improve your own performance in the industry. In the healthcare business, it is helpful to compare your business results with similar businesses such as other hospitals of the same type and size. The physician's office results can be compared to other physicians offices as well. Some reasons for benchmarking are:

- Allows organizations to see where they stand in regard to operational metrics when matched against their competitors and counterparts in the business.
- Assists organizations to understand where they have strengths and weaknesses in their operations.
- Allows organizations to view how much better their competitors can perform in certain metrics and how much opportunity for improvement in their business.
- Helps your organization improve their competitive advantage by stimulating continuous improvement to maintain high performance and competitive standards.
- Can help explain and satisfy customer's needs for quality, cost, product, and services by reviewing industry standards.
- Can be used to establish new goals and commitments by the organization improvement.
- Benchmarking should not just be comparing your healthcare business with national averages; it should involve reviewing the best in class and finding out what they are doing.

Benchmarking sources are widely available from different companies and resources and can be provided free of charge, as part of an association fee, or charge at the cost of service. There are three basic resource categories of benchmarking sources:

Professional associations—Professional associations are great source of benchmarking data. Groups such as the American Medical Association and the Medical Group Management Association are the front-runners of professional associations to publish data for the members. While these are still strongly used associations, most professional associations supply some type of benchmarking data for their members. There are many discipline-specific associations such as the American College of Radiology or the American Academy of Pediatrics that supply benchmarking data specific to their member base.

Government—Federal and state government bodies have been collecting, analyzing, and publishing healthcare-related data for some time to enable healthcare organizations to improve their businesses. Most of the data supplied is to improve the quality of healthcare which in turn improves the financial side as well. The Centers for Medicare and Medicaid is one source that provides healthcare data for use by the public. Most of the data supplied by government agencies is free of charge, but fees may be charged for specific data banks.

Private entities—There has also been a growing number of private businesses in the industry that collect, analyze, and sell financial, operational, and quality data that can be used by healthcare organizations to improve their business. Many of these private entities are consulting firms and financial service companies or have other main businesses in the healthcare sector. These groups are publishing this data to make profits for their company, so there will be a charge for the use of this data. Some groups can be the McKesson, Gallup, Ernst & Young organizations and other similar type organizations.

Benchmarking data can be very useful for healthcare organizations to improve their business. This data can be accessed publicly or privately and can then be free or cost thousands of dollars for the information. When purchasing healthcare benchmarking data, one should be certain that the data requested is useful to the end user. It can be useful to ask for samples of data so they can be certain that they were purchasing the information that is useful to them and their company.

Further Reading

Cleverley W, Cleverley J, Song P. Essentials of health care finance. Sudbury, MA: Jones & Bartlett Learning; 2011.

Finkler S, Ward D. Accounting fundamentals for health care management. Sudbury, MA: Jones and Bartlett; 2006.

Gapenski L, Pink G. Understanding healthcare financial management. Chicago, IL: Health Administration Press; 2011.

Getzen T. Health economics and financing. Hoboken, NJ: Wiley; 2010.

Getzen T. Health economics and financing. Hoboken, NJ: Wiley; 2013.

Huss W, Coleman M. Start your own medical practice. Naperville, IL: Sphinx; 2006.

Keagy B, Thomas M. Essentials of physician practice management. San Francisco, CA: Jossey-Bass; 2004.

Kongstvedt P. Managed care. Boston, MA: Jones and Bartlett; 2004.

Marcinko D, Hetico H. The business of medical practice. New York: Springer; 2011.

Reiboldt J. Financial management of the medical practice. Chicago, IL: American Medical Association; 2011.

Solomon R. The physician manager's handbook. Sudbury, MA: Jones and Bartlett; 2008.

Yousem D, Beauchamp N. Radiology business practice. Philadelphia, PA: Saunders; 2008.

Chapter 9
Budgeting and Variance Analysis

Abstract Budgeting and variance analysis are concepts that may seem to be intimidating, labor-intensive, and confusing for many people. In reality, they are very useful tools in business that are simply our predictions, estimates, and projections of the future of your business. They are not as complicated as some people may think. Budgeting is a process of planning how one expects their business to perform productively and financially in the next period of time. The process budgeting is a prediction of how your business will perform overtime in regard to both income and expenses of your business. The final budget can be very useful to monitor your business over the time period and enable you to make adjustments to stay on course of projections by analyzing variances. Variance analysis is a process to see how well your predictions in the budget came to fruition. Variances in your actual business can be used to make adjustments in your financial and business operations and guide your business to a more successful future.

Budgeting

A budget process can be a good foundation for all the financial activities of a medical business. Budgeting sets a financial plan in terms of productivity, revenue, and expenses for a certain time period, such as the next year. It gives you a chance to look at your business and make predictions of how your business will perform in the future. Most companies budget for a year at a time based on the fiscal reporting year. The actual results of your business can be compared to your budget figures to perform various analyses. This gives businesses the ability to see how the company is performing financially and productively compared to the budgetary goals set forth in the prior year. The following are some of the benefits of a budget:

- Opportunity to reevaluate your business
- Opportunity to review your business potential
- Provides a timely and accurate tool to analyze actual results versus predicted

- Enables the control of future performance
- Helps determine where resources should be allocated
- Provides an early indication of negative variations
- Illuminates signs for future opportunities

The Budget Process

The budget process begins with information gathering and the assembling of the correct people. Some of the people that can be involved in this process are the practice or department administrator, the physician, and the accountant or financial analysts. Documents that should be gathered are as follows:

- Last year's or periods' financial statements
- Productivity reports that show the amount of services provided in the last year to be matched with the financial statements
- Employee and physician productivity reports
- The list of new services for business ventures expected for the coming year
- Contracts or other legal documents showing payment expectations for leases, loans, service agreements, and other future-known financial liabilities
- Bills and statements showing costs for fixed expenses such as gas and electrical, telephone, Internet, and other expenses to run the business
- Some knowledge of outside influences that could affect the budgeting process such as inflation, regulatory changes, taxation changes, competition, demographic considerations, or other side effects

Preparing a Budget

The preparation and completion of a budget involves a number of steps as follows:

Revenue Recognition—The first step is to review the amount of revenue generated last year for each type of service and the number of services associated with that revenue. Last year's income statement is the best place to find the revenue and expenses from the last period of time. In this hypothetical example, a physician's practice or hospital department has five physicians that produced revenues of $5 million based on 16,000 visits in the last year. The average office visit included some ancillary-billed procedures, and the average office visit revenue was $25. The contractual discounts were 25 % of revenue or $6.25 per visit. The net operating revenue was $25 less the $6.25 for contractual discounts, leaving a net operating revenue of $18.75 for each patient visit.

These figures would now be used to predict our next year's revenue projections. The firm has estimated that the number of visits will increase to 17,000, the price per visit will increase to $27, and the contractual discounts are expected to increase to 30 %. Our projections for next year would be as follows: 17,000 times $25 equals revenue of 425,000 for each of the five doctors or $2.125 million total. Expected contractual discounts would be 30 % of 2.125 million or $637,500. The expected net operating revenue would be $2.125 million minus $637,500 or $1,487,500. This is a basic example of the revenue recognition for a budget. Many other factors can come into play, including multiple revenue-generating services in a medical practice for business, additional services, and individual factors for each provider of the business. Hospitals will have each department contribute with revenue inputs into the overall hospital budget. The department budgets will be produced first and then added to the consolidated budget for the hospital.

Expenses

Fixed Expenses—As mentioned in Chap. 4, a fixed expense is an expense that will occur whether or not the business is open or any transactions take place. Examples of fixed expenses are rent, insurance costs, leasing costs, equipment maintenance costs, and other expenses that must be paid. This data is gathered from the last income statement, as well as the invoices, contracts, and legal documents that were gathered previously. The different expenses should be line items and projected out as designated by their documents. If rent for a year is $12,000, then a line item for rent should be added for $1,000 per month and so forth. Physician and nonphysician salaries, wages, and employee expenses such as taxes and benefits can be both a fixed expense and a variable expense. Fixed-salaried employees whose income will not be changed depending on business can be considered fixed expenses and can be estimated in this area.

Variable Expenses—Variable expenses are expenses that only occur when the business is running and performing services. These are normally a fee-per-visit-type charge. A physician visit may use $5.00 in medical supplies during a visit including EKG leads, tongue blades, paper or table, etc. Some other variable expenses may be medical supplies, billing services, and office supplies. These are only incurred when services are performed. The practice plans to see 17,000 office visits next year; then the expected budgeted number for medical supplies during these visits is $5.00 times 17,000 or $85,000. Some employees may only work based on the amount of business occurring. These employees would be a variable expense since their salaries and employment taxes may be different each week. For these employees, estimate the number of hours we expected them to be employed per week increased by the prorated tax and benefit liability percentages.

Other Income and Expenses—The income statement showed us that there are other incomes in the business and expenses that are not related to the actual operations, such as investment income and losses, charitable donations, or other items that increase or decrease the other revenue shown on the income statement.

Final Budget—The budget for the future period should look very similar to the last income statement of the business. The line items should be comparable except for

Buckeye Medical Center
Income Statement
Years Ending December 31, 2012 and 2011

Financial statements in U.S. dollars

	2012	2013 Budget	Change
	(In Thousands)		
Operating Revenue			
Operating Revenue	1,109,822	1,198,608	Increase of services by 8%
Less: Contractual Discounts	410,634	467,457	Increase in contractual of 2%
Net Operating Revenue	699,188	731,151	
Operating Expenses			
Salaries and Wages - Non Physician	221,504	225,934	Increased by 2%
Professional Fees	85,371	90,323	Increased by 8%
Employee Benefits	89,986	91,786	Increased by 2%
Supplies	69,220	73,235	Increased by 8%
Purchased Services	48,454	51,264	Increased by 8%
Facilities	29,995	29,995	fixed
Insurance	11,536	11,536	fixed
Utilities	9,229	9,229	fixed
Interest Expense	8,625	8,625	same
Depreciation and Amortization	41,532	43,138	same percentage of revenue
Bad Debt	13,599	14,623	same percentage of revenue
Other	4,514	4,514	same
Total Operating Expenses	633,565	654,201	
Income From Operations	65,623	76,949	
Non Operating Revenue (Expenses)			
Investment Income (loss)	15,000	12,000	prediction
Community Support and Charity	(55,682)	(57,761)	same percentage of revenue
Other	7,596	7,596	same
Total Non Operating Income	(33,086)	(38,165)	
Net Income (Loss)	32,537	38,785	

Fig. 9.1 Income statement showing actual 2012 results and 2013 budget with change percentages

additions and deletions of services. After the new budget is formed, it should be compared to the previous income statement for verification that the revenues and expenses are comparable to the previous income statement. In other words, if the cost of rent for a year was $12,000 and that number did not increase, then your rent in the new budget should be the same. For demonstration purposes, Fig. 9.1 shows the income statement of Buckeye Medical Center in one column and the projected budget in the next column.

It can be seen from this example that they expect to increase operational revenue by 8 %. In addition to this, salaries and wages are increasing by 2 % due to raises. Many of the building costs are not rising, and depreciation and bad debt are expected to maintain the same ratios to revenue. In nonoperating revenue, investment income is a good guess, but they have a good judgment of what charity will be. They expect the net income to increase by $6,248,000. This will be considered the final budget for approval by the board of directors or trustees.

Variance Analysis

Variance analysis is a comparison of what was predicted and what actually happened in the business in regard to revenue and expenses. The analysis is the examination, interpretation, and investigation of the differences between what was planned and what actually happened. This should not be perceived as a tool to find blame for unfavorable results, but a management control tool to improve unfavorable variances in the future. The results of this analysis should help your company modify or change directions, revise plans, or tighten controllable expenses. A few key points about variance analysis are:

• To be used as a proactive means to explain why variances occurred between the budgeted and actual results of the business.
• A tool to inform the administration of a business or hospital why the actual results of the business are better and worse than expected.
• A resource that enables the business to make changes in a positive direction for future growth and viability.
• A variance analysis should be performed every time the income statement is reviewed, such as a monthly basis.
• Every line of the income statement does not need to be analyzed for variance. One should consider certain parameters for review such as a difference of 5 or 10 % between the actual and budgeted figures. Variances over that specified parameter should be investigated further.
• Variances can be red flagged and watched on a continued basis in the future.
• Various analyses are used to illustrate developing trends.

Reviewing income and expense variances is a very important part of the financial and accounting side of the business. If either the income or expenses of the business vary greatly, the bottom line of the business will be affected in either positive or negative direction. A positive variance is obviously good for a business and negative variance is not so good for a business, but either way, the administrator needs to know why these variances occurred for the future growth and sustainability of the company. Variance analysis is performed by comparing the actual amounts of income or expenses to the budgeted estimates of income and expenses. These variances can be viewed as a dollar amount or percentage difference. The administration should set up rules in regard to which accounts need to be further analyzed for variance based on set parameters. These parameters can be:

• Variances that exceed a certain dollar amount
• Variances that exceed a fixed percentage value difference between the budgeted and actual values
• All variances that display an unfavorable or negative amount
• A combination of one of the three factors above

All variances that match the parameters set by the administration should be reviewed in depth for an explanation of the difference. These variances should be

Buckeye Medical Center
Income Statement
Years Ending December 31, 2012 and 2011

Financial statements in U.S. dollars	January Actual	January Budget	Variance	Percent Change
Operating Revenue		(In Thousands)		
Operating Revenue	88,569	99,884	(11,315)	−11.33%
Less: Contractual Discounts	32,771	38,955	(6,184)	−15.88%
Net Operating Revenue	55,798	60,929	(5,131)	−8.42%
Operating Expenses				
Salaries and Wages - Non Physician	15,524	18,828	(3,304)	−17.55%
Professional Fees	7,127	7,527	(400)	−5.31%
Employee Benefits	7,568	7,649	(81)	−1.06%
Supplies	5,012	6,103	(1,091)	−17.88%
Purchased Services	4,596	4,272	324	7.58%
Facilities	2,500	2,500	0	0.02%
Insurance	1,523	961	562	58.43%
Utilities	756	769	(13)	−1.70%
Interest Expense	688	719	(31)	−4.28%
Depriciation and Amortization	3,598	3,595	3	0.09%
Bad Debt	1,425	1,219	206	16.94%
Other	253	376	(123)	−32.74%
Total Operating Expenses	50,570	54,517	(3,947)	−7.24%
Income From Operations	5,228	6,412	(1,184)	−18.46%
Non Operating Revenue (Expenses)				
Investment Income (loss)	3,500	1,000	2,500	250.00%
Community Support and Charity	(4,201)	(4,813)	612	−12.72%
Other	500	633	(133)	−21.01%
Total Non Operating Income	(201)	(3,180)	2,979	−93.68%
Net Income (Loss)	5,027	3,232	1,795	55.55%

Fig. 9.2 Income statement displaying actual January results, budgeted January amounts, and the variances. Variances also displayed as a percentage of difference, either positive or negative

recorded, discussed with managers and administrators of the business, and tracked for future periods. An action plan to manage this variance should be developed.

Figure 9.1 shows the budget for next year for Buckeye Medical Center. In Fig. 9.2, the yearly budget is broken down to a monthly budget, evenly distributed per month. In reality, many companies budget unevenly throughout the year to account for high points and low points in the yearly cycle. This example will be evenly distributed. The first column shows the actual January income statement numbers and the second column shows the budgeted numbers. The next column shows the positive or negative variance between the budgeted and the actual numbers, and the final column displays this difference as a percentage of change.

The first variances are in the operating revenue. Operating revenue is $11,315,000 under what was expected or 11.33 % off. Contractual discounts were off as well by 15 %. The net operating revenue was down by $5,131,000 or 8.42 %. This would be considered an unfavorable variance, and the company should investigate why the operating revenue was so low. Buckeye should investigate the different parts of the operating revenue such as office visits and ancillary activities to see where the variances are occurring. The doctor's offices visits may be off budget or the ancillary services may be down as well. After the areas of variance are found, the medical facility can put together a plan to correct these variances to be more favorable in the next period.

The variances in the expense section do not look as dramatic as the revenue section. The salary and wages were 17 % below budget. This is actually favorable and could be a sign that the company reduced hours of employees during the month because they may have forecasted reduced revenue during the month and reacted appropriately. Supplies were also down by over $1,000,000 which would be consistent with supplies being a variable expense which would be lower if service revenue is lower. Purchase services were up for the month compared to budget, and it may be a good idea to investigate why these were increased. These are normally known in advance and should not vary much. The same is true for insurance which was almost double the budgeted amount. There could have been a change in contracts, added liabilities, or discontinued coverage. Facilities, utilities, interest expense, depreciation and bad debt, and others were slightly different from budgeted but not of a concern at this time. In total, the expenses were off by almost $4,000,000 or 7 %. This shows that the firm adjusted its resources during a month and reduced those in response to the slowed business. Income from operations was off by $1.1 million or −18 %.

Nonoperating revenue and expenses showed a positive variance of investment income of about $2.5 million. Community support was down slightly and will probably rebound in the next month. In total, the nonoperating revenue had a positive variance of almost $3 million. This positive variance helped the bottom line or net income with a boost of $1.7 million. This is quite interesting since the actual operations of the business lost money and the nonoperations made money, resulting in a positive net income for the company. This occurrence does happen in healthcare businesses, so the administrator needs to pay attention to operations as well as nonoperations.

Further Reading

Cleverley W, Cleverley J, Song P. Essentials of health care finance. Sudbury, MA: Jones & Bartlett Learning; 2011.

Finkler S, Ward D. Accounting fundamentals for health care management. Sudbury, MA: Jones and Bartlett; 2006.

Gapenski L, Pink G. Understanding healthcare financial management. Chicago, IL: Health Administration Press; 2011.

Getzen T. Health economics and financing. Hoboken, NJ: Wiley; 2010.

Getzen T. Health economics and financing. Hoboken, NJ: Wiley; 2013.

Huss W, Coleman M. Start your own medical practice. Naperville, IL: Sphinx; 2006.

Keagy B, Thomas M. Essentials of physician practice management. San Francisco, CA: Jossey-Bass; 2004.

Kongstvedt P. Managed care. Boston, MA: Jones and Bartlett; 2004.

Marcinko D, Hetico H. The business of medical practice. New York: Springer; 2011.

Reiboldt J. Financial management of the medical practice. Chicago, IL: American Medical Association; 2011.

Solomon R. The physician manager's handbook. Sudbury, MA: Jones and Bartlett; 2008.

Yousem D, Beauchamp N. Radiology business practice. Philadelphia, PA: Saunders; 2008.

Chapter 10
Strategic Planning and Business Planning

Abstract Strategic planning is focused on viewing the internal and external environments, discovering opportunities for future business goals, and then setting a plan to accomplish the goals. A business plan is a detailed plan for expansion of services or for a new business venture to include both a conceptual and a financial plan. There are some commonalities among these processes. They all review the history and current status of your company and then look into the future state of your company based on your mission, vision, and goals. The future could include new ideas for expansion, business relationships, and new projects for businesses. Each of these processes will be reviewed with examples, including a business plan for a new venture.

Strategic Planning

Strategic planning is a tool that assists management and effective decision-making. It is a process of assessing your present situation, deciding where you want to be in the future, making a plan of how to get there, and then putting that plan into action.

This process of analyzing, planning, integrating, and then putting into action is detailed in this strategic planning process as shown in Fig. 10.1.

Perform a SWOT Analysis

The SWOT analysis is completed by performing an assessment or audit of the internal and external environments of the company. One of the key considerations of strategic planning is to understand internal (your own organization) strengths and

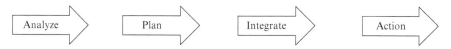

Fig. 10.1 Typical steps in strategic planning process

Strengths	**Weaknesses**
Broad line of services	Limited service line
Wide geographical base	Small geographical base
Good customer satisfaction	Poor customer satisfaction
Good base of physician employees	Limited employed physicians
brand-name recognition	Mediocre reputation
Newer assets	Older and obsolete assets
Good financial management	Poor financial management
Strong management team	Weak management team
Strong purchasing and supply system	Poor purchasing and supply system
Opportunities	**Threats**
Expand service line	Consumer preferences changing
Exploit new targets	encroachment of core business
Expand existing service lines	Competition increasing market share
Expand geographically	Increase of new competitors
Enter new business lines	Changing demographics
Overcome barriers to entry	Changes in the company
Reduce rivalries among competitors	Market is in a slow growth mode
Acquire profitable businesses	Labor costs and unions are increased

Fig. 10.2 SWOT analysis chart

weaknesses as well as external threats and opportunities. Therefore, the four parts of a SWOT analysis are labeled strengths, weaknesses, opportunities, and threats:

- *S*trengths: Traits or characteristics of your business that give you a competitive advantage in the market
- *W*eaknesses: Traits or characteristics of your business that make your business weaker or at a competitive disadvantage to others in the market
- *O*pportunities: Areas of expansion or new services that can be exploited in the market
- *T*hreats: Parts of the environment that can impede the growth and success of your organization or cause negative issues for it as well

An example of a SWOT analysis chart is shown in Fig. 10.2.

Strengths

Strengths are all the positive attributes that your business has, including tangible and intangible assets. Strengths include services that your business does well, the type of resources and assets that you have, and what you do better than your competition does.

One should evaluate each of the companies attributes, including the management, finance, each department, employees, marketing, and organizational structures. Strengths include the positive attributes of your employees, including their education, experience, and background. Other strengths include assets such as equipment, property and plants, goodwill, copyrights and patents, existing customers and vendors, and relationships with outside vendors and businesses.

These strengths should highlight your positives or competitive advantages that you find internally in your company. These strengths will be used to exploit your future goals and objectives. Some strengths may be having the latest robotic surgery technology available or very seasoned employees with great skills and vision.

Weaknesses

Weaknesses are the negative aspects of your business that decrease the strength of your company in areas where you do not have a competitive advantage. These are also tangible and intangible assets in your business. Weaknesses can include limited resources, poor service offerings, lack of experience and education of your employees, lack of technology, or weak assets in regard to plants, properties, and equipment. Weaknesses can be old and dilapidated buildings that need to be replaced or very weak balance sheet items such as very limited short-term cash and securities.

Weaknesses are the negative attributes internal to your business that cause you to have a competitive disadvantage in the market. These are areas where you need to improve in order to be competitive. You should always be honest and transparent when reviewing the weaknesses of your company and look for opportunities for improvement and growth.

Opportunities

The opportunities section reviews the external factors of your market which occur outside the walls of your business but within the market where you work. Opportunities can be seen as needs in the environment and in the market that you are able to fulfill with your current or potential strengths.

Opportunities may be the result of growth in the market, weaknesses of your competitors, the ability to create a new service and implement it, or any technology or service that is not available in your area. Remember, true opportunities are found outside or external to your business. If you have identified "opportunities" that are found inside the organization and within your control, then they should be classified as strengths. An opportunity may be that your competitor does not have any neurosurgeons employed at the time and is lacking a neuroscience business or your company has the opportunity to introduce a new type of radiation therapy into the local market.

Strengths	Weaknesses
Opportunities	Threats

Fig. 10.3 SWOT analysis chart displaying examples of strengths and weaknesses as well as external threats and opportunities

Threats

What are the threats to your business? External threats are situations which you have no control over. Some threats can be unfavorable trends, current and new competitors, price increases from vendors, revenue decreases from insurance and government payers, government regulations, bad economic times, or shifts in consumer demand. This is a good time to put all of your fears from your environment under the SWOT matrix for you to investigate.

The stronger you are in identifying threats in your area, the more able you are to defend or position yourself and to be proactive to mitigate your risks. Some threats may be a large hospital system moving into your area or Medicare reducing payments to physicians by 10 %.

Determine Market Position and Competitive Advantage

After your SWOT analysis, you have a fair understanding of where your medical business stands in regard to your competitors. You should plot these factors on the SWOT matrix in Fig. 10.3 and gain a good visual of these four categories. This will give you a better determination of your market position. You should also plot where you plan to be in the future. From this analysis, the firm should be able to analyze the data and determine some areas for competitive advantage and opportunities for the future. Competitive advantage can be barriers to entry of other firms, protection from government regulations, economies of scale, customer loyalty, or a financial advantage to purchase new technology equipment and grow.

Establish Strategic Objectives or Goals

In this step, opportunities are transformed into goals and objectives. It is recommended to use a SMART goal, which means that your goal should be specific (S), measurable (M), achievable (A), realistic (R), and time bound (T). SMART goals are within your achievable scope and give you a potential for success. A SMART goal may be to hire an orthopedic knee specialist to grow your orthopedic surgery business by 10 % over the next year.

Form a Strategic Business Plan

The strategic business plan is the plan for how the company will progress from the current market state of your business to the obtaining of the goals and objectives. A business plan will be discussed in more detail in the next section.

Gain Management Support

The key to successful strategic plans is the support of upper management and the board of directors or trustees. Without their financial, managerial, and emotional support, your project or business venture has a greater chance of failure. They must approve and commit to all parts of your plan. The best method for getting their support is to provide them with a thorough business plan and sufficient supporting documentation.

Implement, Monitor, and Adjust as Needed

After approval from the management and/or boards of directors, it is time to implement the plan and the business. A plan with ongoing strategy-focused measuring, monitoring, and adjusting will make the strategy successful.

Business Plan

A business plan is a formal statement of your business goals and the plan for achieving those goals. This document will establish the plans in terms of the operational, managerial, marketing, and financial aspects.

Executive Summary

This is normally a one-page summary of your overall business plan. It is the first section of a business plan, but the last part written. It summarizes what and who the company is, what they plan to do, how they plan to get there, and what the financial goals of the plan are. An example of an executive summary is as follows:

Buckeye Medical Center is a fictitious 565-bed health system located in central Ohio serving acute care patients and outpatients in primary and specialized care areas. It opened 25 years and is the leading health system in the area. The administration has performed a SWOT analysis and discovered one of their strengths is their imaging department, especially in the MRI division. This department is a high-revenue and high-quality producer for the hospital. Recently, the FDA has approved a new 3T MRI system with great potential in healthcare. The area market of Buckeye does not have a 3T MRI system yet. Buckeye will purchase a 3T MRI system and locate it in the main hospital. It would be the first 3T MRI system in the area. The system will be installed in the current MRI department as an additional system. The system will cost $2.5 million and will be paid from cash reserves of the hospital. The system should be financially feasible and successful by having a return on investment of 1.2 years and a break-even volume of 3.0 patients per day based on 240 days per year. The marketing department in the hospital has already started an initial marketing plan to advertise and promote the new MRI system in the area. The hospital administration is confident that it can gain volume from both its loyal physician providers and any area providers that do or don't currently refer to the MRI department. A market survey displayed a willingness of these physicians to refer to the new technology.

The actual executive summary should be about one page long, but this provides a good example of what's to be included in it.

Company Information

This includes the makeup of the company, to include some of the following:

- Business structure
- Purpose of company
- For profit or not for profit

- Owners of the corporation
- Nature of the business
- Locations and services provided
- Brief data and other company number of patient visits, surgeries, emergency room visits, etc.
- Any other factual information about the company itself that can help sell your business plan and gain financial support

Description of New Business

This section talks about the project or venture of this business plan and why you wish to pursue this venture. It should start with a brief history about MRI and its uses. It would be explained in this section about the present uses of MRI and the future uses with this new technology. This would detail why a need exists and how this technology would fill the need. It would explain why this project would be successful.

Marketing Plan

The marketing plan is a very important part of any business plan. It talks about the 4Ps of marketing, which are product, price, place, and promotion of your project. The product is a 3T MRI system and the price is the MRI procedure charge of $3,500 per exam. The place is the location (in the MRI department). Promotion is how you will sell your new service to your community in regard to education, advertising, and other marketing vehicles to promote your new business.

Management and Human Resources—This section will discuss the management and human resources, structure, and responsibilities. This section will also list new human resources that will be needed for the success of this plan. An organizational chart showing the reporting structure from the MRI technologist up to the administration should be shown. Finally, any training and education of present and future staff should be described.

Financial Documents and Analysis

The financial documents to be presented in this section are similar to the ones presented in the text including the income statement or pro forma, cash flows, and ratios or financial analysis. The income statement is actually called a pro forma in a business plan. It is very similar to the budget statement discussed in the beginning of this chapter. The revenues and expenses are estimated in relation to your new business project of the new 3T MRI system. The pro forma should only include items related to this project. Generally the pro forma is established for a 3- to 5-year period. The company wants to see how this new venture will produce revenue for the next few years.

Assumptions for the project are always required for the plan so that people know how you made your projections. The assumptions for the new 3T MRI are:

- Cost of system and related equipment is 2.5 million dollars.
- Construction cost will be $300,000.
- System will be purchased with current cash.
- Straight-line depreciation will be used for 7 years or $357,000/year.
- Revenue per exam is $3,500/exam.
- Contractual discounts will be 60 % of revenue.
- Number of procedures will be 6/day in year 1 and then increase in years 2–5 by 2/day.
- Year will be counted as 240 days of business based on 20 average days per month (weekdays only, less holidays, less service and maintenance days, and less training days).
- Two technologists will operate the system—cost is $30.00/per hour.
- Benefits and taxes for employees are 20 % of wages.
- Salaries increase 2 % per year and maintenance will be $110,000 for years 2–5.
- Supplies per exam will be $25.00/exam.
- MRI contrast and medical supplies are estimated at $100.00 per case.
- Professional interpretations are $75.00 per exam.
- Facilities expenses are $1,000/month increasing by 3 % per year.
- Utilities are $500.00/month increasing by 3 % per year.
- Insurance is $400/month.
- Interest expense will be $850/month.
- Bad debt is 1 % of revenue.
- Others are $500.00/month.

The pro forma for this project is shown in Fig. 10.4.

This MRI project looks to be a success with the pro forma. All of the assumptions are entered into the pro forma, and the bottom line shows that this will produce positive net incomes throughout the 5-year plan. MRI is always a high-revenue generator and can normally produce strong financials. The next part of the financial analysis is to look at the cash flow for the project. Cash flow is the revenue minus expenses for a business plan like this. The cash flows for this project are in Fig. 10.5.

As you can see, only the first year does not produce positive cash flow since more money was spent for the purchase of the MRI system in that year than flowed in from using it. Over the course of 5 years, there is positive cash flow of $9.8 million.

Sometimes in a cash flow statement like this, there is an increased flow of cash in the final year of the project from selling the machine at its salvage value. In the assumptions it was noted that the life of this project is 7 years, but the pro forma is

Buckeye Medical Center
Pro Forma - MRI Project
January 1, 2014 - December 31, 209

Financial statements in U.S. dollars

		2014	2015	2016	2017	2018
Operating Revenue			(In Thousands)			
	Number of Exams	1,440	1,920	2,400	2,880	3,360
	Operating Revenue	5,040,000	6,720,000	8,400,000	10,080,000	11,760,000
	Less: Contractual Discounts	3,024,000	4,032,000	5,040,000	6,048,000	7,056,000
	Net Operating Revenue	2,016,000	2,688,000	3,360,000	4,032,000	4,704,000
Operating Expenses						
	Salaries and Wages - Non Physician	124,800	127,296	129,842	132,439	135,088
	Professional Fees	108,000	144,000	180,000	216,000	252,000
	Employee Benefits	24,960	25,459	25,968	26,488	27,018
	Supplies	36,000	48,000	60,000	72,000	84,000
	Facilities	12,000	12,240	12,485	12,734	12,989
	Insurance	4,800	4,800	4,800	4,800	4,800
	Utilities	6,000	6,120	6,242	6,367	6,495
	Interest Expense	10,200	10,200	10,200	10,200	10,200
	Depriciation and Amortization	357,000	357,000	357,000	357,000	357,000
	Bad Debt	20,160	26,880	33,600	40,320	47,040
	Other	6,000	6,000	6,000	6,000	6,000
	Total Operating Expenses	709,920	767,995	826,138	884,348	942,629
	Income From Operations/Net Income	1,306,080	1,920,005	2,533,862	3,147,652	3,761,371

Fig. 10.4 Pro forma for MRI project

CASH FLOWS

3T MRI System	Year 1	Year 2	Year 3	Year 4	Year 5	Total
Initial Capital Investment	(2,800,000)					(2,800,000)
Additional Revenue	2,016,000	2,688,000	3,360,000	4,032,000	4,704,000	16,800,000
Additional Expense	709,920	767,995	826,138	884,348	942,629	4,131,030
Expected Cash Flow	(1,493,920)	1,920,005	2,533,862	3,147,652	3,761,371	9,868,970
Cummulative Cash Flow	(1,493,920)	426,085	2,959,947	6,107,599	9,868,970	9,868,970

Fig. 10.5 Cash flow stream for MRI project

only for 5 years. Therefore, salvage value of $250,000 for the MRI system will not be part of this cash flow.

As part of this plan, there are financial ratios and formulas that are required by most institutions to beautify financial success of a project. Some of the most important ones are the return on investment (ROI), net present value (NPV), internal rate of return (IRR), break-even analysis, and the payback period.

Ratios

Return on Investment (ROI)—The ROI is an important element in a project's financial analysis. It is a predictor of expected profitability. ROI is a very popular financial metric to analyze the financial prediction of new projects, capital acquisitions, investments, and other initiatives. This is one of the first financial analysis calculations that is reviewed by financial officers in a corporation for new project viability. This projection number can make or break a project's chance of being approved by management.

ROI is sometimes called the measure of profitability. The ROI can tell a firm how much revenue you will receive for your investment, does the revenue outweigh the costs, and is a project worth it for the firm in the long run. ROI is calculated as a ratio or percentage. The calculation is as follows:

ROI = (Net Income – Investment Costs)/Investment Costs

For this project, the ROI is as follows:

$$ROI = \left(1,306,080 + 1,920,005 + 2,533,862 + 3,147,652 + 3,761,652 - 2,800,000\right)$$
$$/2,800,000 = 352\%$$

This is a very positive predictor for this project with a relatively high ROI. The ROI is good for prediction purposes but may be less trustworthy in complex projects. Therefore, one should not solely rely on the ROI to make a project decision.

Net Present Value (NPV)—The NPV is a profitability measure using a discounted cash flow to see what the value of this project is as of today. This measure looks at the inflows and outflows of cash during the life of the project and determines the present value of the cash flow. In other words, how much are all cash flows worth today at current interest rates. If the NPV is positive, then the project will be profitable. The higher the NPV, the better the chances of a profitable and successful project. If the NPV is negative, then the project is unprofitable and it may not move forward. The actual calculation for an NPV is as follows:

$$NPV = I_0 + \frac{I_1}{1+r} + \frac{I_2}{\left(1+r\right)^2} + \ldots + \frac{I_n}{\left(1+r\right)^n}$$

where I_0 = initial investment, I = income amounts each year, r = discount rate, and N = number of years of investment.

This can be calculated easier using the NPV formula in excel.

You would enter the range of cash flows over the 5 years and the present interest available in the market. A 6 % interest rate will be used for this example. The NPV of this project is $7,143,753.19. This means that if the company had all cash flows in their hands today with the current interest rates, then the project is worth all over $7 million. This also is a good indicator of success for the project.

Internal Rate of Return (IRR)—A third profitability measurement is internal rate of return or IRR. The IRR can be considered for the discounted cash flow rate of return. This is the interest rate that would produce a NPV of $0. In other words, how much does the company have to discount all of the inflows and outflows of the project over the 5 years to have a net present value of zero? The higher the projects IRR, then the more desirable it is to take on the project. Calculation for the IRR is

$$NPV = \sum_{n=0}^{N} \frac{C_n}{(1+r)^n} = 0$$

where n=period, C=cash flow, N=total number of periods, and NPV=net present value.

For this project, you should use the excel formula for IRR while using the range of cash flows and an interest figure of 10 %. The IRR for the MRI project is 65 % which signals a very strong project.

Payback Period—This is a calculation that shows how long it will take for the cash flows to pay for this investment. In other words, how long will it take until the cash flow equals the cost of the investment in the project? The calculation is

Payback period$=(p-n)/p+$ny

where p=the cash flow value in the first positive cash flow period=$1,920,005, n=the cash flow value in the last negative cash flow period=1,493,920, ny=the last period which shows a negative cash flow=1

Payback period$=(1,920,005-1,493,920)/1,920,005+1=1.2$ years. It will take 1.2 years to pay back the investment of this project. Most companies like this number to be under 2 or 3 years.

Break-Even Analysis

Breakeven is a financial calculation which displays the revenue or volume of services that need to be performed in order to break even. Breakeven is the point at which revenues equal expenses. Until the break-even point is reached, the company project will be unprofitable and losing money. Once the break-even point is reached, the project will make money. There are two ways to look at breakeven. One way is to look at as the number of units to sell to break even the amount of sales in dollars. Before we can calculate breakeven, we need to determine three factors:

- Fixed expenses
- Variable expenses
- Sales

For calculation of breakeven, we use fictitious numbers from Widgets, Inc., and determine how many widgets need to be sold in order to break even.

Fig. 10.6 Sample fixed
expenses for Widgets, Inc.

Widgets, Inc.
Fixed Expenses Per Year

Administrative Costs	$ 6,000
Rent	$ 2,500
Salaries	$ 40,000
Office Expenses	$ 1,000
Insurance	$ 500
Dues And Subscriptions	$ 1,000
Equipment Leases, Payments On Loans	$ 50,000
Depreciation	$ 5,000
Advertising	$ 14,000
	$ 120,000

Fig. 10.7 Sample variable
expenses for Widgets, Inc.

Widgets, Inc.
Variable Expenses Per Year

Direct or Raw Materials	$ 5.00
Sales Commissions	$ 1.00
Production Supplies	$ 2.50
Credit Card Fees	$ 0.20
Packaging Supplies	$ 0.50
Shipping Costs	$ 0.60
	$ 9.80

Fixed Expenses—A fixed expense (F) is an expense that does not vary with sales. It has to be paid if you sell one unit or 50 units. Examples of fixed expenses are:

- Administrative costs
- Rent
- Salaries
- Office expenses
- Insurance
- Dues and subscriptions
- Equipment leases and payments on loans
- Depreciation
- Advertising

The sample fixed expenses for Widgets, Inc., are shown below in Fig. 10.6.

Variable Expenses—A variable expense varies with each sale. If you sell 0 units, then you incur no variable costs. As you sell units, you start incurring a variable cost per unit. Below are examples of variable expenses:

- Direct or raw materials
- Sales commissions
- Production supplies
- Credit card fees
- Packaging supplies
- Shipping costs

The sample variable expenses for Widgets, Inc., are shown below in Fig. 10.7.

Sales—The next item needed is the net sales price. The net sales price for this calculation is the actual selling price less any discounts or contractual arrangements. In this example, a widget has a selling price is $25.00 and the average discount is $3.00. The net sales price is $22.00 per widget.

The *variable cost percentage per unit* also needs to be determined. We look at variable sales as a percent of sales price. If your net sales price (NS) is $22.00 and the variable cost per unit (V) is $9.80, then the variable cost per unit as a percentage of sales (VS) is $9.80/$20.00 or 45 % of sales.

Formulas

There are two formulas for breakeven based on units and sales volume in dollars:

Break-Even Units = Total Fixed Costs/(Net Sales Revenue – Variable Cost Per Unit)

$$S = F / (NS - V)$$

Break-Even Sales = Fixed Expenses + Variable Expenses as a Percentage of Sales

$$S = F + VS$$

Break-Even Units = Total Fixed Costs/(Net Sales Revenue – Variable Cost Per Unit)
$S = F/(NS - V)$
$S = 120,000/(22 - 9.80) = 9,836$
9,836 widgets must be sold to break even.

Break-Even Sales = Fixed Expenses + Variable Expenses as a Percentage of Sales
$S = F + VS$
$S = 120,000 + 0.45S$
$S - 0.45S = 120,000$
$0.55S = 120,000$
$S = 120,000/0.55 = \$218,181.82$
$218,181.82 in sales is needed to break even.

Profit Break-Even Predictions

A firm can determine the amount of sales or units needed to make a certain profit. If Widgets, Inc., wishes to make a profit of $100,000, then what is their sales units and sales revenue needed?

The same formulas apply except the profit (P) amount is added to fixed cost amount:

Break-Even Units = Total Fixed Costs/(Net Sales Revenue – Variable Cost Per Unit)

$S = F + P/(NS-V)$

$S = 120,000 = 100,000/(22-9.80) = 18,033$

18,033 widgets must be sold to make $100,000.

Break-Even Sales = Fixed Expenses + Variable Expenses as a Percentage of Sales

$S = F + VS$

$S = 655,760 + 0.15S$

$S - 0.15S = 655,760$

$0.85S = 655,760$

$S = 655,760/0.85 = 771,482$

$771,482 in sales is needed to break even.

MRI Real-Life Example: Breakeven

In our MRI project, how many MRIs per day must be performed in order to break even? The revenue after contractual discounts, fixed costs, and variable cost per unit can be found in our assumptions as is shown in Fig. 10.8. For variable expenses as a percentage of sales, if the net sales price (NS) is $1,400.00 and the variable cost per unit (V) is $214, then the variable cost per unit as a percentage of sales is $214/1,400 or 15 % of sales:

Break-Even Units = Total Fixed Costs/(Net Sales Revenue – Variable Cost Per Unit)

$S = F/(NS-V)$

$S = 655,760/(1,400-214) = 553$

553 MRIs must be performed to break even.

Break-Even Sales = Fixed Expenses + Variable Expenses as a Percentage of Sales

$S = F + VS$

$S = 655,760 + 0.15S$

$S - 0.15S = 655,760$

$0.85S = 655,760$

$S = 655,760/0.85 = 771,482$

$771,482 in sales is needed to break even.

In summary, this chapter has examined the budgeting process followed by the variance analysis to be used with the budget. The second half of the chapter reviewed the strategic planning process including a business plan and all of the essential parts, including a more detailed pro forma and profitability analysis. The tools learned in this chapter will be used throughout your career if you are involved in administration and business planning. Now that you have the financial reporting, analysis, budgeting, and business planning completed, the next few chapters will discuss insurance, managed care, and business structures with an integration of the tools learned in this chapter.

Break-Even Assumptions

Description	Values	Calculation	Revenue/Expense Amount
Revenue after Contractual Discounts			
Revenue per exam is $3500/exam	3500		
Contractual discounts will be 60% of revenue	0.6	$3500 * (1 - 40\%)$	$ 1,400.00
		Revenue after Contractual Discounts	**$ 1,400**
Fixed Costs			
2 technologists will operate the system – cost is $30.00/per hour	30/hr, 2040 hr/year, 2 technologists	30*2040*2	$ 124,800
Benefits and taxes for employees is 20% of wages	20% of wages	20% * 124,800	$ 24,960
Service and Maintenance will be $110,000 for years 2-5	110000/year	110000*1	$ 110,000
Facilities expenses are $1000/month increasing by 3% per year	1000/month	1000*12	$ 12,000
Utilities are $500.00/month increasing by 3% per year	500/month	500*12	$ 6,000
Insurance is $400/month	400/month	400*12	$ 4,800
Interest Expense will be $850/month	850/month	8500*12	$ 6,000
Other is $500.00/month	500/month	500*12	$ 10,200
Depreciation will be 7 years straight line or $357,000/year	357,000/year	357,000*1	$ 357,000
TOTAL		**Total Fixed Costs/year**	**$ 655,760**
Variable Expenses			
Supplies per exam will be $25.00/exam	25/exam	25*1	$ 25
MRI Contrast and medical supplies are estimated at $100.00 per case	100/exam	100*1	$ 100
Professional interpretations are $75.00 per exam	75/exam	75*1	$ 75
Bad Debt is 1% of revenue	1% per exam	1% * 1400	$ 14
TOTAL		**Total Variable Costs/exam**	**$ 214**

Fig. 10.8 Break-even assumptions for MRI real life example

Further Reading

Cleverley W, Cleverley J, Song P. Essentials of health care finance. Sudbury, MA: Jones & Bartlett Learning; 2011.

Dahl O. Think business! Phoenix, MD: Greenbranch; 2007a.

Finkler S, Ward D. Accounting fundamentals for health care management. Sudbury, MA: Jones and Bartlett; 2006.

Gapenski L, Pink G. Understanding healthcare financial management. Chicago: Health Administration Press; 2011.

Getzen T. Health economics and financing. Hoboken, NJ: Wiley; 2010.

Getzen T. Health economics and financing. Hoboken: Wiley; 2013.

Hacker S. The medical entrepreneur. [U.S.?]: Nano 2.0 Business Press; 2010.

Harbin T. The business side of medicine. Minneapolis: Mill City Press Inc.; 2013.

Huss W, Coleman M. Start your own medical practice. Naperville, IL: Sphinx; 2006.

Keagy B, Thomas M. Essentials of physician practice management. San Francisco: Jossey-Bass; 2004.

Kongstvedt P. Managed care. Boston: Jones and Bartlett; 2004.

Marcinko D, Hetico H. The business of medical practice. New York: Springer; 2011.

Reiboldt J. Financial management of the medical practice. Chicago, IL: American Medical Association; 2011.

Solomon R. The physician manager's handbook. Sudbury, MA: Jones and Bartlett; 2008.

Yousem D, Beauchamp N. Radiology business practice. Philadelphia: Saunders/Elsevier; 2008.

Dahl O. Think business! Phoenix, MD: Greenbranch; 2007b.

Chapter 11
Healthcare Insurance

Abstract Insurance is protection to cover individuals against some type of loss or risk. Common types of insurance include automobile, home, and business insurance. These insurances provide the consumer with a protection against some type of risk such as an automobile accident or home damage. Health insurance was invented to protect the consumer against health issues or risks because the cost of healthcare prevention, diagnosis, and treatment can be very expensive. Most people are unable to pay for their healthcare needs with their current incomes and need assistance to pay for medical services. The concept of health insurance has been around for 150 years and has evolved into a major part of the healthcare business. Health insurance is available in some manner to all citizens of the United States and can be provided by private insurance companies or federal and state governments. Healthcare insurance can be funded by employers, by state and federal governments, or by individuals. The healthcare insurance system needs to be understood by healthcare professionals to provide quality care for their patients and receive the proper reimbursement for their services. This can involve some type of collaboration between insurance providers, payers, and beneficiaries.

What Is Health Insurance?

Health insurance is a contract with a company that provides payment for medical services including prevention, sicknesses, and injuries. This insurance can be paid for by your employer, by your federal or state government, or by specific individuals. It protects people from having to pay for the full cost of medical services when someone is sick or injured. There are many different types of healthcare insurance which have been changing throughout its history. Insurance policies differ in what and who they cover, the amount of out-of-pocket money the patient has to pay, limits of payment, and treatments or services that are covered.

History of Health Insurance

The history of health insurance goes back to the mid-1800s and has evolved over time. Here are some of the key activities and events that have shaped the healthcare insurance market that we have today:

1847—Massachusetts Health Insurance Company issues sickness insurance (Barton 2010).

1850—Travelers Insurance Company offered medical insurance to consumers (Barton 2010).

1910—Montgomery Ward and Co. starts a group insurance program (Mcdonnell 2002).

1910—National Convention of Insurance Commissioners created the first law regulating health insurance (Mcdonnell 2002).

1929—The first employer-paid health insurance program is accredited to school teachers at Baylor University Hospital in Dallas Texas (Barton 2010).

1930—Blue Cross was established as an insurance company (Barton 2010).

1939—The Revenue Act of 1939 established employee tax exclusion for workers' compensation claims and benefits (Mcdonnell 2002).

1943—Henry Kaiser sets up first prepaid insurance plan (TMCI 1988).

1947—The Taft-Hartley Act was a major push for employer-paid insurances and established health benefits as a condition of employment for which labor was entitled to negotiate (Barton 2010).

1948—The McCarran-Ferguson Act gives states power to regulate insurance (Mcdonnell 2002).

1954—The Revenue Act of 1954 excludes employers' insurance contributions from taxation (Mcdonnell 2002).

1965—President Johnson passes Title XVIII and Title XIX of the Social Security Act to start Medicare and Medicaid.

1973—The Health Maintenance Organization (HMO) Act of 1973 requires all employers with over 25 employees to offer an HMO option to their health benefit plans.

1986—The Consolidated Omnibus Budget Reconciliation Act of 1985 (COBRA) requires employers with 20 or more employees to offer continued health coverage to terminated employees and dependents (Mcdonnell 2002).

1996—The Health Insurance Portability and Accountability Act (HIPAA) of 1996 sets national nondiscrimination and "portability" standards for individual health insurance coverage (Mcdonnell 2002).

1997—The Balanced Budget Act of 1997 (BBA) creates the Medicare+Choice program and Children's Health Insurance Program (CHIP) (Mcdonnell 2002).

2003—The Modernization Act of 2003 expands the Medicare law to include prescription drugs.

2010—The Patient Protection and Affordable Care Act (PPACA) extends insurance to more than 30 million uninsured people by expanding Medicaid, creating healthcare insurance exchanges, and mandating employer insurance and providing federal subsidies to help lower- and middle-income Americans buy private coverage.

Key Health Insurance Terms and Definitions

The following terms and definitions will help you understand the insurance industry:

Beneficiary—Anyone who is covered for medical services under an insurance plan.

Payer—The company or person that actually pays for medical services.

Provider—The physician, hospital, or medical company providing medical services.

Benefits—The medical services covered by the insurance plan.

Premium—The amount paid each month or year for the healthcare insurance.

Co-payments—Payment defined in the insurance policy and paid by the insured person for each medical service at the time of service. A physician's office may require a $20 co-payment at the time of visit or a $10 co-payment for prescription drugs at the pharmacy.

Fee-for-service—This is a payment for services rendered specific to that service. A fee will be paid to healthcare providers specifically for each service (like an office visit, test, or procedure).

Coinsurance—In the fee-for-service type of payment system, the patient may be responsible for a portion of the bill charges. Oftentimes, the patient is responsible for 20 % of the bill charges, while the insurance company will pay for their 80 %.

Deductibles—The amount of expenses that must be paid out of pocket before an insurer will pay any expenses. A patient may have a $200 deductible for his insurance plan. After the patient pays for $200 worth of services out of their pocket, then the insurance will start paying for any expenses occurred after that time. Deductibles are renewed or start at $0 for every new insurance premium year.

Maximum out-of-pocket expenditure—The maximum amount of money paid by the beneficiary for medical services in a calendar year. The patient may have to make co-payments and deductibles until the amount is reached. After this amount is reached by the patient, then the insurance company will pay a hundred percent after this point. A hypothetical maximum out of pocket may be $3,000. After the patient reaches $3,000 in out-of-pocket costs, then all other expenses will be totally paid by the insurance company.

Preexisting conditions—These are conditions that can make a person a higher risk to an insurance company. A preexisting condition may be a patient with cancer or a heart condition, and their insurance may be hard to find or expensive looking for an insurance company.

Coordination of benefits—This occurs when someone has two insurance plans such as a husband and wife who both work and both have insurance coverage at work. Both insurance plans look to ensure that the appropriate insurance company pays for services rendered.

Gatekeeper—A physician who manages a patient's healthcare services, coordinates referrals, and helps control healthcare costs by screening out unnecessary services.

Comprehensive policies—A comprehensive policy is one that includes most medical services from inpatient services to outpatient services, medical testing, medical equipment, mental health, and prescription drugs. Normally the only exclusions are experimental procedures and therapies.

Major medical or hospital surgical policies—This is a specific insurance type in which the benefits provided are those illnesses requiring hospitalization. Any services or treatments required outside of a hospital stay are normally not included.

Catastrophic coverage policies—These are policies which are intended to cover patients after the lifetime limit has been reached. These policies are in addition to the normal health insurance policy.

Disease-specific policies—Specialized insurance policies that only cover specific diseases such as heart disease, cancer, or other serious illnesses.

Medigap policies—These are supplemental or voluntary commercial insurance policies that cover the difference between amounts covered by Medicare and amounts not covered by Medicare.

Types of Healthcare Insurance Coverage

Insurance types can be distinguished between private insurance and public insurance. Private insurance includes any insurance plans paid by the employer, patient, or other funding individual or institution. Public insurance includes any federal or state government-sponsored programs.

Private Insurance

Private healthcare insurance is also referred to as voluntary health insurance because it is not mandated. Private insurance is funded by groups or individuals that choose to have insurance. This can include employers, individuals, or representatives of individuals who want to pay for their health insurance.

Indemnity Plans Versus Managed Care Plans—Group insurance, individual private insurance, and self-insurance are considered indemnity plans. There are no contracts between the insurer and providers. It is a medical plan that reimburses the patient and/or provider as expenses are incurred. In managed care plans, there are contracts between the insurer and the provider of services, and expenses are paid at predetermined, discounted, or capitated rates.

Group Insurance—Group insurance is normally obtained through an organization such as the employer, a union, or a professional organization. There are a substantial number of people in this type of group, which distribute the risk and cost of the group among the members. Group insurance is normally paid for by your employer. In most situations, the employee is expected to pay a part of the health insurance along with their employer. Major companies which provide group health insurance are Blue Cross Blue Shield, Aetna, and UnitedHealthcare.

Individual Insurance—Not all employers provide health insurance benefits to their employees. In situations when people cannot obtain healthcare benefits through their employer, then they must seek individual insurance plans on their own. They can still obtain insurance through the companies mentioned above, but the risk is not spread across a large number of people as it is in group insurance and the premiums, deductibles, and coinsurance are much higher for these individuals.

Self-Insurance—Some larger companies like to act as an insurance company and assume the risk of their employees. In a situation where the employer is self-insured, that employer will pay the medical claims incurred by their employees. The employer normally buys a reinsurance or risk insurance to protect itself against the potential risk of high losses or high medical claims by its employees.

Managed Care Plans—The insurance company contracts with healthcare providers in an effort to control costs, access, and quality of healthcare services provided to its beneficiaries. Managed care plans are where the insurer has incentivized goals to reduce costs and increase quality and access to healthcare services. Examples of managed care organizations are health maintenance organizations (HMOs), preferred provider organizations (PPOs), and point of service (POS) plans. Managed care will be described in more detail in the next paragraph.

Public Insurance

Public financing began in 1965 when President Johnson signed the Social Security Act of 1965. This act enabled Medicare and Medicaid to be initiated as programs for the elderly, disabled, and indigent. Public insurance can be defined as health insurance that is financed by the federal or state government and is of little or no costs to beneficiaries. Medicare and Medicaid are the two largest government-sponsored insurance programs in the United States. Besides Medicare and Medicaid, other government programs are programs for the military, veterans, and injured workers and programs for Native Americans.

Medicare—Medicare is also referred to as the Title XVIII of the Social Security Act and is the second largest public health insurance, caring for three groups of people: (1) people 65 years of age and older, (2) disabled individuals entitled to such security benefits, and (3) people who have end-stage renal disease (CMS 2013). Medicare is a federally funded program operated by the Centers for Medicare and Medicaid Services (CMS), which is a branch of the US Department of Health and Human Services (DHHS). Medicare has four different parts to it: A, B, C, and D.

Part A—Medicare part A is also known as hospital insurance. It covers:

- Hospital care
- Skilled nursing facilities
- Nursing home care
- Hospice care
- Home health services
- Non-covered services including long-term care, custodial services, and personal convenience services (Medicare 2013)

Medicare part A is funded by the payroll tax of 1.45 % from the employee and 1.45 % from the employer (Shi and Singh 2012). Some beneficiaries of 65 years of age or older do not have to pay a premium if they meet the Social Security Administration's qualifications, while those who don't qualify will have to pay a monthly premium.

Part B—Medicare part B is also known as supplemental medical insurance. This is a voluntary program with a premium that provides coverage for physician visits and outpatient services. Part B covers:

- Physician services
- Emergency department visits
- Outpatient surgery
- Diagnostic tests
- Laboratory tests
- Outpatient physical, occupational, and speech therapy
- Outpatient mental health services
- Part-time home healthcare
- Ambulance services
- Renal dialysis
- Artificial limbs and braces
- Blood transfusions
- Organ transplants
- Medical equipment and supplies
- Rural health clinic services
- Annual physical exams
- Preventive care services such as mammography, cancer screening, glaucoma screening, pap smears, flu shots, etc.
- Non-covered services including dental services, hearing aids, eyeglasses, and medical services not related to an injury or treatment

Part B is financed approximately 25 % from the enrollees and 75 % from federal treasury funds. There is a deductible and coinsurance in addition to the monthly premium (Shi and Singh 2012).

Part C—Medicare part C is known as *Medicare Advantage* and is the "managed care" Medicare service. The Balanced Budget Act of 1997 authorizes the *Medicare + Choice Program,* which became effective on January 1, 1998. This allowed private insurance to expand their Medicare managed care-type program.

Medicare + Choice was renamed *Medicare Advantage* in 2003. Medicare Advantage offers additional benefits compared to basic Medicare and has lower out-of-pocket costs. Medicare recipients are able to choose a Medicare Advantage Plan yearly between November 15 and December 31, with the benefits starting January 1 of the next year.

Part D—Medicare part D is the prescription drug benefit. This is a voluntary program and requires a monthly premium for the coverage. This program can be added to any Medicare beneficiary. It is also offered as a stand-alone prescription drug program or as a Medicare Advantage Prescription Drug Program which is available through managed care organizations that are participating in Medicare part C. There is one challenge of the Medicare part D program, which is called the "doughnut hole." The basic level of Medicare pays for 75 % of the cost of drugs until the total payments for a beneficiary reaches $2,840. After this point, the beneficiary reaches the doughnut hole and must pay 50 % of the cost of brand-name drugs or 7 % on generics until the beneficiary has spent $4,550 out of pocket. After that, the patient leaves the doughnut hole area and enters the catastrophic level and only pays a small portion of the drug cost. This doughnut hole challenge is addressed in the Affordable Care Act of 2010 which will be discussed later.

Medicaid—Medicaid is also known as Title 19 of the Social Security Act and is the largest provider of public health insurance in the United States. It is jointly funded by the state and federal governments, and its purpose is to cover the medically indigent. The following categories of individuals are automatically eligible under federal Medicaid guidelines: (1) families with children receiving support under the temporary assistance for needy families (TANF) program, (2) people receiving supplemental security income (SSI), (3) children and pregnant women with income at or below 133 % of the federal poverty level, (4) and other areas defined by federal law. Medicaid services include the following.

Mandatory Benefits

- Inpatient hospital services
- Outpatient hospital services
- EPSDT: early and periodic screening, diagnostic, and treatment services
- Nursing facility services
- Home health services
- Physician services
- Rural health clinic services
- Federally qualified health center services
- Laboratory and x-ray services
- Family planning services
- Nurse-midwife services
- Certified pediatric and family nurse practitioner services

- Freestanding birth center services (when licensed or otherwise recognized by the state)
- Transportation to medical care
- Tobacco cessation counseling for pregnant women
- Tobacco cessation

Optional Benefits (Dependent on Each State's Discretion)

- Prescription drugs
- Clinic services
- Physical therapy
- Occupational therapy
- Speech, hearing, and language disorder services
- Respiratory care services
- Other diagnostic, screening, preventive, and rehabilitative services
- Podiatry services
- Optometry services
- Dental services
- Dentures
- Prosthetics
- Eyeglasses
- Chiropractic services
- Other practitioner services
- Private duty nursing services
- Personal care
- Hospice
- Case management
- Services for individuals aged 65 or older in an institution for mental disease (IMD)
- Services in an intermediate care facility for the mentally retarded
- State plan home and community-based services—1915
- Self-directed personal assistance services—1915
- Community First Choice Option—1915
- TB-related services
- Inpatient psychiatric services for individuals under age 21
- Other services approved by the secretary (Medicaid 2013)

Medicaid is financed by both the state and federal governments. The federal government will pay approximately 50–75 % of the total Medicaid costs based on the wealth of the states (Tate 2012). The average federal contribution is 57 % with the average state contribution being 43 % (Tate 2012). The Medicaid program is operated by the state governments. The recipients for Medicaid must qualify based on assets and income which must be below the threshold levels established by each state. This threshold is based on the relation to the federal poverty level.

The threshold from the states falls around the 133 % markup federal poverty level and will be above or below this number depending on each state.

Children's Health Insurance Program (CHIP)—This is also known as the State Children's Health Insurance Program (SCHIP). CHIP was formed under Title 21 of the Social Security Act in 1997. This program benefits children whose parents have income too high to be eligible for Medicaid, but the income is too low to afford private insurance. CHIP provides benefits for the children and not the parents. CHIP covers children in families with incomes below 200 % of the federal poverty level as long as the child is not covered under another insurance program (Medicaid 2013). This program is funded and operated similarly to the Medicaid program in which the federal and state partner in the financing, with the federal government paying approximately 65 % of the cost (Medicaid 2013). The state government operates the CHIP program, and the Affordable Care Act has extended the program until October 1, 2015 (Medicaid 2013).

Program of All-Inclusive Care (PACE)—The PACE program involves the expansion of the Medicare and Medicaid programs. PACE provides comprehensive long-term services to Medicare and Medicaid enrollees. The service enables enrollees to receive care at home rather than at a nursing home. Eligibility requirements include:

- Aged 55 or older
- Living in the service area of a PACE organization
- Eligible for nursing home care
- Able to live safely in the community (Medicaid 2013)

PACE benefits include all benefits provided for Medicare- and Medicaid-covered services programs and are provided primarily in an adult day health center and by in-home and referral services as needed by the enrollee (Medicaid 2013). An inter-disciplinary committee ensures that the comprehensive medical and social needs of each participant are met. PACE providers are paid capitated rates from Medicare and Medicaid.

TRICARE—TRICARE is the title of the *Military Health Services System (MHSS)* that provides healthcare benefits for military personnel, veterans, and their dependents. TRICARE offers three programs for its enrollees: HMO, PPO, and a fee-for-service program. All active-duty members are automatically enrolled in the HMO program at no cost. The PPO program and the fee-for-service program both require enroll-ment and a fee. TRICARE has three main features: (1) it is recently managed to facilitate administration of the program, (2) it is structured in the same format as managed care, and (3) it is able to combine the medical resources of the army, navy, and air force and combines the internal medical services of the MHSS and the civil-ian healthcare professionals and networks. TRICARE has four regions, including the north, south, west, and overseas regions. Each region provides oversight over their geographical area and their health plan administration, manages regional con-tracts, supports commanders at military medical facilities, engages providers for areas not served by military hospitals and clinics, and finances regional initiatives to optimize and improve delivery of healthcare (TRICARE 2013). A couple of drawbacks with TRICARE are that there are a limited number of network providers in rural areas, challenges to providing rehabilitative services to injured soldiers, covering national guard and reserve personnel who alternate between active and inactive duty, and ensuring that they have a sufficient amount of providers and facilities to care for the beneficiaries.

Veterans Health Administration (VHA)—The VHA was formally called the *Veterans Administration (VA)* and is a department of the US government. The VHA is now a division of the VA and manages the health services branch. The VHA operates 152 medical centers and approximately 1,400 community-based outpatient clinics, community living centers, vet centers, and domiciliaries. These healthcare facilities and the more than 53,000 independent licensed healthcare practitioners provide comprehensive care to more than 8.3 million veterans each year (VHA 2013). VHA Medical Centers provide a wide range of services including surgery, critical care, mental health, orthopedics, pharmacy, radiology, physical therapy, audiology, speech pathology, dermatology, dental, geriatrics, neurology, oncology, podiatry, prosthetics, urology, and vision care. Some medical centers also offer advanced services such as organ transplants and plastic surgery (VHA 2013).

The VHA program was originally intended to treat veterans with war-related injuries and re-rehabilitate soldiers with those injuries. The mission was expanded to include most of the care needed by veterans of low income. There are eight categories of enrollment for the VA which include categories for disabilities, prisoners of war, low income, and veterans exposed to potential disease-causing situations such as radiation and herbicide exposure. The VA is a tax-financed agency and provides most of its care through government-salaried physicians in government facilities. The budget is appropriated by the president and approved by congress. The VHA also operates a program called CHAMP. This program covers dependents of disabled veterans and survivors of veterans who died in the line of duty, died from service-related conditions, or were currently disabled at the time of death.

Indian Health Services (IHS)—IHS is a division of the *Department of Health and Human Services (DHHS)* and provides comprehensive medical and healthcare services to members of federally recognized American Indian and Alaska Native tribes and their descendents. The IHS provides a comprehensive health service delivery system for American Indians and Alaska Natives who are members of the 566 federally recognized tribes across the United States (HIS 2013). Services include medical and dental care, health promotion and disease prevention programs, substance abuse programs, maternal and child health, sanitation, and nutrition. They have their own system of hospitals, health centers, and health stations.

Workers' Compensation—Workers' compensation is a state-administered program. Employers are financially liable for the full cost of injuries and illnesses that are a result of working conditions. There are four categories of workers' compensation benefits: (1) cash payments for lost wages, (2) payment for medical treatments, (3) indemnification for loss of occupational capacity and skills, and (4) survivor death benefits. While worker's compensation is operated by the state government, it is funded by the employer either through private insurance, a state fund in which employers contribute, or self-insurance. Most workers' compensation programs are operated under the same principles as managed care.

US Public Health Service

The US Public Health Service was established in 1798 as the Marine Hospital Service as it was signed into the law by President John Adams (Sultz and Young 2014). This first law provided services for seamen who are sick or disabled. This was followed by the creation of the Public Health Service Commissioned Corps. in 1889. In 1902, the Marine Hospital Service's name was changed to Public Health and Marine Hospital Service and again changed to the official present name of US Public Health Service in 1912 (Sultz and Young 2014). The US Public Health Service was a department of the US Treasury Department from its inception until 1939 when it became a member of the Federal Security Agency. In 1953, the US Public Health Service became part of the newly created Department of Health, Education, and Welfare. This department was later renamed as a Department of Health and Human Services (DHHS) in 1979. The DHHS continues to be the government owner for the US Public Health in its mission to protect and promote the provision of health and other human services to vulnerable populations. Currently, the DHHS includes over 300 separate programs. These are some of the agencies of the DHHS:

National Institutes of Health (NIH)—This organization was established in 1887 and is the world's premier medical research organization and includes separate health institutes, the National Center for Complementary and Alternative Medicine and the National Library of Medicine. Their mission is to promote research toward preventing and curing diseases. This department supports over 3,000 research projects for writing medical conditions (Sultz and Young 2014).

Food and Drug Administration (FDA)—This agency has the responsibility of ensuring the safety of foods, human and veterinary products, electronic products, cosmetics, pharmaceuticals, biological products, and medical devices.

Centers for Disease Control and Prevention (CDC)—The mission of this agency is to protect health and promote quality of life through the prevention and control of disease, injury, and disability. This agency is primarily responsible for protecting American public's health through the monitoring of disease trends, investigations of outbreaks of health in injury risks, and implementing illness and energy control with preventative measures. The CDC's focus areas are health impact, customer focus, public health research, leadership, globalization, and accountability. It was created in 1946.

Indian Health Service (HIS)—This agency provides healthcare services to Native Americans and Alaska Natives that live in the United States. Their mission is to raise the physical, mental, social, and spiritual health of American Indians and Alaska Natives.

Health Resources and Services Administration (HRSA)—This agency is responsible for programs serving low income, uninsured, and medically underserved populations. Their funds are used for comprehensive primary and preventive services through community-based health centers nationwide. They also support maternal and child health programs in underserved communities. This agency has six bureaus: primary healthcare, health professions, healthcare systems, maternal and child, the HIV/AIDS Bureau, and the Bureau of Clinician Recruitment and Service.

Substance Abuse and Mental Health Services Administration (SAMHSA)—This agency works to improve the quality and availability of substance abuse prevention programs, addiction treatment, and mental health services. Its funding is through federal block grants. It also provides a variety of grants to state local communities for substance abuse, mental health service needs, and AIDS.

Occupational Safety and Health Administration (OSHA)—This agency was established in 1970 with a mission to govern a safe and healthy environment and workplace. Some of the programs created by OSHA are the Hazard Communication Standards, the Medical Waste Tracking Act, and the Occupational Exposure to Blood-Borne Pathogen Standards.

Agency for Healthcare Research and Quality (AHRQ)—This is the agency that supports research to improve the quality of health, reduce healthcare costs, improve safety of patients, address medical errors, and address access to service challenges in our country. They also sponsor and conduct research for evidence-based information and healthcare outcomes in regard to quality, cost, uses, and access. The focus of the agency-supported research is in healthcare cost and utilization, information technology, disaster preparedness, medication safety, healthcare consumerism, prevention of illness, and special needs population.

Department of Homeland Security (DHS)—This division was established in 2002 as a result of the 9/11 terrorist attack in 2001. They are responsible to manage catastrophic events and coordinate efforts at all government levels to ensure emergency preparedness in regard to bioterrorism, chemical and radiation emergencies, explosions, natural disasters, severe weather, and disease outbreaks.

Centers for Medicare and Medicaid Services (CMS)—This agency was formally known as the Health Care Financing Administration. This program administers Medicare and Medicaid programs. It also administers the Children's Health Insurance Program (CHIP) in our country.

Administration for Children's Families (ACF)—This division administers over 60 programs to promote the economic and social well-being of families, children, individuals, and communities. It also administers the state/federal welfare program, temporary assistance for needy families, national child support enforcement, and Head Start program. Finally, it provides funds to assist low-income families with child care expenses, supports the state programs and adoption assistance foster care, and funds child abuse in the plastic violence problems.

Administration on Aging (AoA)—This agency is the advocacy agency for older persons. This agency is the largest provider of home- and community-based care for older people. Their mission is to develop cost-effective and efficient system for long-term care that helps the elderly maintain health, dignity, and social health in our homes and communities (Niles 2011). This program assists older citizens to remain in their homes and support them with services such as Meals on Wheels. The program is operated through regional offices to plan, coordinate, and develop community-level systems of services so that the older individuals are able to meet their needs.

Agency for Toxic Substances and Disease Registry (ATSDR)—This agency was created in 1985, and its mission is to protect the public against harmful exposures and disease-related exposures to toxic substances (Niles 2011). They are responsible for determining the human health effects associated by toxic exposures, preventing continued exposures, and combining and associating human health risk.

Further Reading

Barton P. Understanding the U.S. health services system. Chicago, IL: Health Administration Press; 2010.

Buchbinder S, Shanks N. Introduction to health care management. Burlington, MA: Jones & Bartlett Learning; 2012.

Cleverley W, Cleverley J, Song P. Essentials of health care finance. Sudbury, MA: Jones & Bartlett Learning; 2011.

Cms.gov. Medicare Program – General Information – Centers for Medicare & Medicaid Services. (Online) http://www.cms.gov/Medicare/Medicare-General-Information/MedicareGenInfo/index.html. Accessed 3 Sept 2013.

Finkler S, Ward D. Accounting fundamentals for health care management. Sudbury, MA: Jones and Bartlett; 2006.

Huss W, Coleman M. Start your own medical practice. Naperville, IL: Sphinx; 2006.

Ihs.gov. About IHS – Indian Health Service (IHS). (Online) http://www.ihs.gov/aboutihs/. Accessed 4 Sept 2013.

Kongstvedt P. Managed care. Boston: Jones and Bartlett; 2004.

Management V. About VHA – Veterans Health Administration. (Online) http://www.va.gov/health/aboutVHA.asp. Accessed 4 Sept 2013.

Marcinko D, Hetico H. The business of medical practice. New York: Springer; 2011.

Mcdonnell K. A brief history of managed care. Washington, DC: Employee Benefit Research Institute; 2002. http://www.ebri.org/publications/facts/index.cfm?fa=0302fact (e-book).

Medicare.gov. Medicare.gov: the official U.S. government site for Medicare. (Online) http://www.medicare.gov/. Accessed 3 Sept 2013.

Medicaid.gov. Medicaid Benefits|Medicaid.gov. (Online) http://www.medicaid.gov/Medicaid-CHIP-Program-Information/By-Topics/Benefits/Medicaid-Benefits.html. Accessed 3 Sept 2013.

Medicaid.gov. Program of All-Inclusive Care for the Elderly (PACE)|Medicaid.gov. (Online) http://www.medicaid.gov/Medicaid-CHIP-Program-Information/By-Topics/Long-Term-Services-and-Support/Integrating-Care/Program-of-All-Inclusive-Care-for-the-Elderly-PACE/Program-of-All-Inclusive-Care-for-the-Elderly-PACE.html. Accessed 3 Sept 2013.

Niles N. Basics of the U.S. health care system. Sudbury, MA: Jones and Bartlett; 2011.

Reiboldt J. Financial management of the medical practice. Chicago, IL: American Medical Association; 2011.

Shi L, Singh D. Delivering health care in America. Sudbury, MA: Jones & Bartlett Learning; 2012.

Shi L, Singh D. Essentials of the U.S. health care system. Burlington, MA: Jones & Bartlett Learning; 2013.

Solomon R. The physician manager's handbook. Sudbury, MA: Jones and Bartlett; 2008.

Sultz H, Young K. Health care USA. Burlington, MA: Jones & Bartlett Learning; 2014.

Tricare.mil. About us. (Online) http://www.tricare.mil/Welcome/AboutUs.aspx. Accessed 4 Sept 2013.

TMCI. A brief history of managed care. Boston, MA: Tufts Managed Care Institute; 1988. http://www.thci.org/downloads/briefhist.pdf (e-book).

Yousem D, Beauchamp N. Radiology business practice. Philadelphia, PA: Saunders/Elsevier; 2008.

Chapter 12
Managed Care

Abstract Managed care is a contractual relationship between the beneficiary, the insurance provider, and the provider of services in order to control costs, increase access, and increase quality of care. The goal is to achieve efficiencies in the delivery of healthcare services, control utilization of medical services, and negotiate the price of services with providers. Managed care has been a growing system in our country for over 30 years and has been the single most dominant force to transform the delivery of healthcare since 1990. As of 2011, 99 % of all workers enrolled in employer-sponsored healthcare insurance plans are enrolled in some type of managed care program (Shi and Singh, Essentials of the U.S. health care system, 2013). All private- and public-sponsored health insurance plans including Medicare and Medicaid offer some form of managed care program. Health maintenance organizations were the first dominant type of managed care followed by point of service plans and preferred provider organizations. Each methodology of managed care will differ according to the provider, delivery of services, payment mechanisms, and risk. This chapter will outline the different managed care structures and their similarities and differences.

Managed Care Defined

Managed care is a philosophy or methodology to manage and control all parts of healthcare including financing, insurance, delivery, and payment:

Financing—Premiums negotiated as part of a contract between employers and the managed care organizations (MCOs). This is generally a fee per member per month (PMPM).

Insurance—The MCO will collect premiums for insuring enrollees and function as an insurance company. The MCO will find facilities to provide all healthcare services required by the enrollees. The MCO will pay for all benefits of their covered population.

R.V. Bucci, *Medicine and Business: A Practitioner's Guide*,
DOI 10.1007/978-3-319-04060-8_12, © Springer International Publishing Switzerland 2014

Delivery—Unlike the fee-for-service model, the MCO makes arrangements with providers of healthcare services such as physicians, clinics, hospitals, and other healthcare companies to provide services to its enrollees. As part of the contract, the MCO will use different methods to manage the utilization of the healthcare services. In some instances, the MCO will employ some physicians and operate its own facilities.

Payment—The two largest types of reimbursement methods are capitation and discounted fees-for-service. Under managed care, the provider will be paid either a capitated rate for all services required or a discounted fee-for-service model where individual services are paid a preset amount as used.

History of Managed Care

The philosophy and characteristics of managed care have been around for a very long time (Shi and Singh 2007). The roots of this ideology can be traced back to the period between 1850 and 1900. At that time, the railroad, mining, and lumber industries provided employees with healthcare services, and the employers directly contracted with a physician to provide the services at a "per rate per worker." The insurance program started by the Baylor University Hospital in Dallas Texas in 1929 was a PMPM rate of payment and was the first evidence of a capitated program (Shi and Singh 2011). In 1932, the Committee on the Cost of Medical Care was formed to research and establish economic solutions in healthcare services. "After 5 years of work, it recommended a system where (1) medical services were provided by physician groups, (2) costs were distributed over persons and time using an insurance program, (3) funds and services dedicated to disease prevention were increased and (4) community agencies coordinated medical care services" (Ross 2002). Following this, the Kaiser Permanente plan was developed in 1933 in order to take care of construction, shipyard, and steelworkers (Kaiser 2013). The Kaiser Permanente plan became publicly available in 1945 and stands today as one of the largest not-for-profit healthcare plans in the United States with 9.1 million members (Kaiser 2013). Managed care grew slowly until 1973 when the Health Maintenance Organization Act was signed into law by President Nixon. This Act authorized $375 million in funding for HMO expansion in the United States and required all businesses with 25 or more employees to offer an HMO health plan option to their employees. Over the next three decades, managed care grew exponentially, and new versions of managed care organizations started to appear besides HMOs, including provider-sponsored organizations, point of service plans, physician hospital organizations, and exclusive provider organizations.

Reason for the Existence of Managed Care—The following factors influenced and promote the evolution and existence of managed care in the United States:

- Increased life expectancy of US citizens
- Increased population of 65 years of age and older
- Constant introduction of medical technology and equipment

- Upward spirals of cost and expenditures and healthcare
- No control of the amount of charges from healthcare institutions and physicians
- No control in the amount of healthcare services ordered by providers
- Increased self-referral from practitioners
- Lack of methods to monitor the appropriate use of inpatient and outpatient services

Attributes of Managed Care—All managed care companies have the following commonalities:

- Relationships with healthcare organizations/providers in order to provide healthcare services to its members
- Established utilization criteria for use of its services
- Predicts and measures cost control
- Financial incentives for the use of providers and facilities
- Varying amounts of risk for overutilization and overspending
- Promote health improvement and disease prevention

Managed Care Utilization Control Methods—There are three methods that MCOs use to effectively control utilization and monitor the use of services:

1. *Predetermination*—Services are required to be preapproved before the enrollees have the service completed. If the services are not preapproved, then the patient will be liable for all charges. A medical expert determines medically necessary for each given case. This determination attempts to ensure that only medically necessary services are actually approved and provided.
2. *Location*—The MCO determines the most appropriate place or types for services to be provided while maintaining the standard levels of quality. For instance, an MCO will designate a certain location for surgeries or may pay for generic drugs as opposed to brand-name drugs.
3. *Review*—Experts for the MCO will intervene in patient's medical treatments by reviewing the current plan of action and then recommend or change the future plan of action for the patient. They standardize the services and treatment plans for all patients.

Types of Managed Care Plans

There are many kinds of organizations that can fit under the term of managed care. This section lists some of the different models, but keep in mind that these models are constantly changing and evolving. There are four main characteristics which can be observed in all managed care plans:

- Provider type and relationship
- How and where services are delivered
- Payment structure
- Risk sharing

Each type of plan will be discussed in reference to these four characteristics.

Prepaid Group Practice (PGP)—This is the earliest type of managed care model that was recommended as part of the 1932 Report on the Committee on the Cost of Medical Care (NCBI 2013). This committee was a self-formed committee to study medical care economics. Insurers, employers, and other parties would contract with physicians or physician groups to provide a predetermined set of services to a specified population for a fixed price. Kaiser Permanente was an early example of a PGP in the 1930s.

Provider type and relationship—Limited to network of physicians or providers that are contracted.

How and where services are delivered—Services are limited to those contracted physician providers at their office locations.

Payment structure—Capitated payments for specified services.

Risk sharing—No risk sharing; the risk is solely bore by the physicians providing care.

Health Maintenance Organizations (HMOs)—While the PGP is considered the first type of managed care product available in the United States, many feel that the HMO is actually the original and first managed care organization. HMOs began to appear in 1970s and grew rapidly after the passing of the Health Maintenance Organization Act of 1973. The focus of HMOs is prevention and screening services to maintain health and prevention and early detection of disease.

Provider type and relationship—Limited to network of physicians or providers that are contracted. Gatekeepers are used in the system.

How and where services are delivered—Services are limited to those contracted at the provider's locations. Specialty services currently available upon referral.

Payment structure—Mostly capitated payments to providers for specified services with some point of service.

Risk sharing—The risk is shared among the providers of care and the HMO.

There are four models of HMOs.

Staff Model HMO—In this model, the HMO employs all of its salaried physicians. These positions are typically paid fixed salaries with bonuses based upon physicians' productivity and HMO profitability. These physicians are solely employed by the HMO. Normally the HMO contracts with local area hospitals for inpatient services. While this choice of HMO makes it easier to control practice patterns of providers, it must employ a large and wide variety of physicians to support a large member base. For the patient, they have a limited choice of physicians which can be a major disadvantage. This has been the least popular type of HMO.

Group Model HMO—Group model HMOs contract with a single multispecialty group practice in hospitals to provide comprehensive health medical services to the enrollees. The group practice in the situation is not limited to the HMO and can take care of non-HMO patients. The physician group is paid a capitated rate for any and all services provided to its members. This lessens the HMO's control over utilization to a certain extent but offers the patients a wider range of physicians and hospital services than the staff model.

Network Model HMO—This model is similar to the group model, but the HMO will contract with multiple physician groups as opposed to one. These providers are usually paid for in a fee-for-service payment-type situation as opposed to a capitated rate. This model usually works in large populations where the members will be widespread in the services at multiple locations. While this expands the patient's choice of physicians and hospitals, it lessens the utilization control of the providers. A primary care physician in a situation is responsible for providing all physician services and is responsible for reimbursement of any outside referrals that the position makes.

Independent Practice Association (IPA)—This is the popular form of HMO. It has allowed smaller physician groups and independent practices to participate in the HMOs. The IPA is a separate legal entity from the HMO. The IPA will contract with physicians independently or in a group; and payments to providers are a fee-for-service model or capitated model. There is often a risk sharing involvement with the physicians where they are withheld a certain percentage of payments. An average of 15 % can be held in a risk pool to be used if the services utilized by the members are more than expected or budgeted. If this risk is not used, then it is normally returned to the providers as a form of bonus. The IPA then contracts with the HMO to provide services for all of its members. This system shifts the utilization control and contracting from the HMO to the IPA. The HMO does share some risk with the IPA group. One major disadvantage for the HMO is the possibility of the IPA discontinued the contract and removing all of its physicians from the HMO. This would leave the HMO without providers to care for its patients.

Why Did the HMO Methodology Fail?

Kaiser Permanente is one of the only large HMOs left in existence. HMOs were around for some time, but did not captivate the healthcare market like many thought. Some of the reasons HMO did not last are:

- Consumers did not want to be told where to go for services. They want free choice.
- Consumers want to be a part of their medical plan and not told to follow a utilization-driven management plan.
- Patient could be at a medical care disadvantage due to limited treatment options.
- Patients complained about services being denied and referrals refused.
- Difficulty in sharing risk with providers.
- Adversarial stance by HMOs with hospitals and physicians.
- Failure to deliver perceived quality.

- Extremely expensive when compared to true insurance.
- Conflicts of interest inherent in HMOs with physicians receiving bonuses for reduced services.
- HMO philosophy morphed into other types of fee-for-service plans.

Preferred Provider Organization (PPO)—PPOs grew out of the model of the HMO and changed the managed care industry. PPOs offered out-of-network options for the enrollees so that they would not be limited to the closed panel of HMO providers. PPOs became popular in the 1990s. The enrollees could choose in-network preferred providers with whom the PPO had established contracts, or they could use out-of-network providers and pay higher copayments and deductibles which increased their out-of-pocket costs. The providers could be contracted independently or as part of a network system. An *exclusive provider organization (EPO)* is a type of PPO, but the enrollees must use the providers within the PPO exclusively. They are able to see patients outside of the network but will be responsible for the total cost of the services. The PPOs make arrangements with in-network providers and negotiate discounted fee-for-service arrangements. Negotiated arrangements with hospitals included diagnosis-based charges, bundled charges for services, and discounted fee-for-service payments.

Provider type and relationship—Providers included in contracted network providers as well as noncontracted out-of-network providers.

How and where services are delivered—Services can be performed with both in-network and out-of-network providers.

Payment structure—In-network providers are paid at discounted fee schedules, diagnosis-based payments, or bundled payments. Out-of-network providers are paid at the same level as in-network, and the patient is responsible for the balance.

Risk sharing—There is no risk sharing. All risk is with the PPO.

Physician Hospital Organization (PHO)—These organizations include physician hospitals, surgical centers, and other medical providers who contract with a managed care organization to provide a full range of services. This is very similar to a PPO, but the hospitals and physicians form a joint venture and contract directly with a managed care organization. This PPO is paid by the MCO and provides hospital and physicians medical services for the beneficiaries.

Provider type and relationship—Providers included in contracted network providers in the PHO.

How and where services are delivered—Services can be performed with both in-network and out-of-network providers.

Payment structure—In-network providers are paid at discounted fee schedules, diagnosis-based payments, or bundled payments. Out-of-network providers are paid at the same level as in-network, and the patient is responsible for the balance.

Risk sharing—There is no risk sharing. All risk is with the MCO.

Point of Service Plans (POS)—This plan is a combination of the best of the HMO features and the best features of a PPO. With this combination, the POS plans are able to use some utilization control while allowing patients to have a wider range of providers of choice. The HMO feature used in a POS plan is capitation and risk sharing with providers along with a gatekeeper utilization control. The PPO feature of a POS allows patients to choose in-network and out-of-network providers. Although these plans are popular in the late 1990s, their popularity has decreased over time.

Provider type and relationship—Enrollees can use both in-network and out-of-network providers.

How and where services are delivered—Services can take place at any in-network or out-of-network provider. There is unrestricted use of specialty services.

Payment structure—There is a combination of capitation and fee-for-service.

Risk sharing—The risk is shared among the providers of care and the managed care organization.

Provider-Sponsored Organizations (PSO)—These are healthcare organizations that form their own MCO. The PSOs offer health insurance and health services to populations in the region. They are both the managed care organization and the provider of healthcare services. They bypass the normal insurance-type companies and contract directly with employers and other purchasers of insurance plans. They are similar to an IPA, but the PSO assumes all risk for the beneficiaries.

Provider type and relationship—Corporation formed of both physicians and hospitals.

How and where services are delivered—Services are limited to those of the PSO company.

Payment structure—Fee-for-service or capitation.

Risk sharing—The risk is all with the PSO.

Medicare and Medicaid Managed Care

Medicare Managed Care

The Balanced Budget Act of 1997 created the Medicare + Choice program that enabled Medicare enrollees to use managed care services. In 2003, the Medicare prescription drug improvement and modernization act renamed the program Medicare Advantage (MA). There are three types of MA plans: (1) coordinated care plans that have contracted providers; (2) medical savings accounts (MSA), which are the Medicare version of a consumer-directed plan; and (3) private plans that model after the traditional Medicare. Part D prescription plans can be sold on a stand-alone basis.

Medicaid Managed Care

Medicaid managed care has been around for approximately 15 years and has been the result of federal legislations aimed at uninsured children. The Balanced Budget Act of 1997 helped the programs expand. Medicaid managed care programs are the responsibility of each individual state and are still financed by both the state and federal governments.

Further Reading

http://www.ncbi.nlm.nih.gov/pmc/articles/PMC1658442/. Accessed 10 Sept 2013.

Barton P. Understanding the U.S. health services system. Chicago, IL: Health Administration Press; 2010.

Buchbinder S, Shanks N. Introduction to health care management. Burlington, MA: Jones & Bartlett Learning; 2012.

Cleverley W, Cleverley J, Song P. Essentials of health care finance. Sudbury, MA: Jones & Bartlett Learning; 2011.

Huss W, Coleman M. Start your own medical practice. Naperville, IL: Sphinx; 2006.

Finkler S, Ward D. Accounting fundamentals for health care management. Sudbury, MA: Jones and Bartlett; 2006.

Ncbi.nlm.nih.gov. "Final Report" of the committee on the costs of medical care. (Online) Kongstvedt P. Managed care. Boston: Jones and Bartlett; 2004.

Marcinko D, Hetico H. The business of medical practice. New York: Springer; 2011.

Niles N. Basics of the U.S. health care system. Sudbury, MA: Jones and Bartlett; 2011.

Reiboldt J. Financial management of the medical practice. Chicago, IL: American Medical Association; 2011.

Ross J. The Committee on the Costs of Medical Care and the Einstein Quarterly. http://www.einstein.yu.edu/uploadedFiles/EJBM/19Ross129.pdf. 2002; 129–34.

Shi L, Singh D. Delivering health care in America. Sudbury, MA: Jones & Bartlett Learning; 2012.

Shi L, Singh D. Essentials of the U.S. health care system. Burlington, MA: Jones & Bartlett Learning; 2013.

Sultz H, Young K. Health care USA. Burlington, MA: Jones & Bartlett Learning; 2014.

Xnet.kp.org. History of Kaiser Permanente|Kaiser Permanente News Center. (Online) http://xnet.kp.org/newscenter/aboutkp/historyofkp.html. Accessed 5 Sept 2013.

Chapter 13
Payment Methods

Abstract Providers of medical services are paid or reimbursed under many different methods and structures. When payments are made by anyone but the beneficiary of the medical plan, it is defined as a third-party reimbursement or third-party payment. This chapter will discuss the different methods and types of payments by private insurers, public insurers, and managed care organizations. A clear understanding of how payments to providers is made can help the healthcare administrator determine which methods of payment are best for the company and will help enable them to negotiate contracts with insurance companies and managed care organizations for their business. Two types of reimbursement will be discussed in this chapter, namely, prospective reimbursement and retrospective reimbursement. The payment methods to be discussed will be bundled payments, capitation, fee-for-service, value system based, fee schedule, and others. Each of these payment methods is calculated in a different manner, and the effects upon payment to the provider will vary accordingly. This chapter will review the common methods of reimbursement to payers including hospitals, physicians, ancillary services, and other types of providers.

Key Definitions

Third-party payer—The first and second parties are the patient and the provider of services. A third party is when someone else besides the first and second parties pays for the services. A private or public insurance payer would be considered third parties.

Charge—The fee set by a provider for the service.

Rate—The amount paid by a third-party provider.

Fee schedule—A list of charges and the rates paid for these charges set by the insurance company.

R.V. Bucci, *Medicine and Business: A Practitioner's Guide*,
DOI 10.1007/978-3-319-04060-8_13, © Springer International Publishing Switzerland 2014

Claim—Services are rendered and the provider files a bill or claim with third-party payer.

UCR—The usual, customary, and reasonable amount to be paid for services rendered. This is the rate which insurers determine to be appropriate.

Contractual allowance—The difference between the charge and what is considered UCR by the insurance provider. A healthcare provider may charge $100 for a service. The third-party payer determines that the UCR for that service is $60. The $40 balance represents a contractual allowance that is to be written off.

Balance billing—The amount of payment left to be paid by the beneficiary after the third party has paid their rate and the contractual allowance has been deducted from the charge. This is normally the amount of deductible or co-payment that the beneficiary is responsible for.

Retrospective Reimbursement

Under a retrospective reimbursement plan, the amount of reimbursement is determined after the services have occurred. This offers a minimal amount of risk to the providers in most cases. The following are methods used under the retrospective reimbursement methodology:

Fee-for-service charges—The provider will be paid a separate payment for each medical service rendered to a patient. The providers of healthcare services are paid at 100 % of the submitted charges. This method of payment is very uncommon now. There is virtually no financial risk for the providers. Insurance companies rarely pay full charges for services.

Discount percentage of charges—Healthcare organizations offer third parties a discounted fee-for-service schedule in return for sending it to a large amount of patients. Typically a hospital may offer an insurance organization a certain percentage of discounts from all of its charges.

Cost—The healthcare organization is reimbursed at the "cost" of the healthcare services. The organization will have to first determine the actual costs involved in providing services. A simple office visit will incur costs of the receptionists, nurse, doctors, facility expenses, supplies, etc. The cost does include a factor for profit. After determination, the cost may be expressed as a percentage of charges. An office visit may actually cost the practice $25 per visit, and the actual charge is $100.00. The cost of charges would then be considered 25 %. The facility will be paid at the rate of $25 per visit or 25 % of charges.

Cost plus percentage—The provider will be paid the cost as determined above plus an add-on percentage to be used for future growth, new services, or other developmental opportunities. The provider will be paid a rate that is based on the cost to provide the service plus. As related to the cost payment, the facility would be paid at the cost of $25 per visit or 25 % of charges, plus 5 % for a total of $30 per visit or 30 % of charges.

Performance-based reimbursement—In this method, the organization is reimbursed on the basis of quality measures, patient satisfaction measures, outcome measure, and other quality measures determined by the insurance provider. The third-party payer uses the assessment of measures and determines the payment. This is a very unpopular method of payment for providers since it involves more risk than the other methods.

Prospective Reimbursement

Under a prospective reimbursement method, the reimbursement is agreed upon and contracted before services are actually provided. These are the reimbursement methods used by MCO:

Per diem—The reimbursement paid on a per hour, per day, or other time period. This is used for physician payments, for work time worked, and for hospitals where the patient's care is paid in a certain amount for each day the patient is an inpatient.

Per diagnosis—The amount paid in respect to each diagnosis. In this situation, it is predetermined that the medical provider will be paid a certain amount of dollars determined by the patient's diagnosis. A patient may enter the hospital with a hernia for surgery to repair the hernia. The hospital will pay one predetermined amount for surgery and reimburse the healthcare provider that amount no matter how many procedures or amount of care is utilized for that patient. The healthcare provider is at risk in a diagnosis-related payment methodology since it may expend more resources and services than can be paid for with the preset amount.

Bundled payments for hospital and physician services—A fixed amount paid by managed care organizations for treatment of patients by multiple providers. The payment is to be shared among all providers. If a physician in a hospital is involved in the treatment of the patient, then they must determine what proportion of the total reimbursement each physician will get from the managed care organization.

Fee schedule—A list made up displaying all services provided with an associated procedure code and related charge.

Capitation—Based on an agreement between a healthcare provider and the insurer, the provider is paid a fixed amount per member per month (PMPM) in exchange for complete healthcare coverage for their beneficiaries during the time coverage. By accepting this type of coverage, the provider has accepted to cover all healthcare needs of all beneficiaries. This can be quite risky for the healthcare provider since a group of beneficiaries may have some catastrophic healthcare issues that require more healthcare resources than anticipated.

Prospective payment system (PPS)—This is a method of Medicare reimbursement which is a predetermined fixed amount. This payment rate is based on the classification system of that service (e.g., diagnosis-related groups (DRG) for inpatient hospital services). CMS uses separate PPSs for reimbursement for acute inpatient hospitals, home health agencies, hospice, hospital outpatient, inpatient psychiatric facilities, inpatient rehabilitation facilities, long-term care hospitals, and skilled nursing facilities.

Physician Reimbursement

There are a multitude of different types of physician payments based upon the payer organization, specialty, location, physician employment structure, and state and federal laws. Physicians can be paid in three different methodologies—salary-based, non-risk, and risk-based models:

Salary based—The following are ways a physician is paid by salary arrangements:

- Fixed salary—Paid a certain amount in fixed time period and is not dependent on performance.
- Performance-adjusted salary—Salary that is based on the amount and quality of work performed.
- Per time basis—Paid on a per time period method.
- Group practice share—Income based on arrangement with group compensation agreements. This is a contractual amount that depends on the physician's contracted salary amount plus any bonuses based on company profits.
- Others—There are other creative types of arrangements that can be made as well.

Non-Risk Payments

- Fee-for-service
- Usual and customary (UCR)
- Discount percentage of charges
- Fee schedule
- Relative value scale (RVS)
- Resource-based relative value scale (RBRVS)

Risk-Based Payments

- Capitation
- Fee-for-service with risk pool withholds
- Budgeted PMPM

Resource-Based Relative Value Scale (RBRVS)—The Medicare reimbursement schedule uses this methodology. This is a pay scale to reimburse physicians that was created by the Omnibus Budget Reconciliation Act of 1989. The CMS initiated this program to develop a new method of reimbursement that is more effective than the current methodologies used. The goal was to determine the physicians based on key metrics of physicians work, costs associated with maintaining a practice, and opportunity costs. This physician work included any time spent before, during, or after procedure. This work was transformed into a measurable unit called the relative value unit (RVU) and is based upon the time, skill, and intensity it takes a physician to provide that service. RVUs are established for each type of service that is identified by current procedural terminology or CPT codes. The physician fee schedule is developed by a complex calculation that takes into account the RVUs for each CPT code along with factors including overhead for the physicians practice, malpractice insurance adjustments, and geographical cost variations. The final product for this calculation is called the Medicare fee schedule which is updated and published every year. State Medicaid programs have implemented similar fee schedules unique to each state for the payment of physician reimbursement levels. Each state's calculation is unique to that individual state.

Hospital-Based Payment Systems

Inpatient Reimbursement

- Straight charges
- Discount percentage of charges
- Per diem
- Diagnosis-related charges (DRG)
- Percent of Medicare
- Case rates
- Capitation

Diagnosis-Related Groups (DRGs)—In 1982, congress passed the *Tax Equity And Fiscal Responsibility Act (TEFRA)* which focused on Medicare cost control. Part of the bill included a mandate for hospitals to be paid or reimbursed along the lines of a Prospective Payment System (PPS) where reimbursement rates were established in advance for conditions. Based on this PPS, Medicare reimburses a fixed amount per admission and per diagnosis, based on the patient's diagnosis-related group or DRG. In essence, DRG rates are simply bundled payments for each diagnosis. The patient being admitted for coronary heart disease would be reimbursed at a higher level than someone being admitted with a fractured femur in the leg. This DRG reimbursement amount covers any and all medical services provided by the inpatient facility to care for that patient under their diagnosis. DRG reimbursement amounts will differ in different geographical areas, urban versus a rural hospital location, teaching versus nonteaching hospital, and a factor based on the share of low-income patients and that geographical location. For this type of system, a hospital can make more money by reducing the amount of healthcare services allocated for each patient with their perspective diagnosis. The DRG reimbursement system has forced hospitals to minimize length of inpatient stay and implement utilization control methods for testing procedures. Similarly, each state Medicaid program has implemented its own DRG-type reimbursement system which will be different with each state reimbursement calculation methodology.

Outpatient Services at Hospital

- Straight charges
- Discount percentage of charges
- Percent of Medicare
- Case rates
- Capitation
- Ambulatory surgery center (ASC) rates under HOPPS
- Ambulatory Payment Classifications (APC) (DRGs for outpatient services provided at hospital)
- Ambulatory Payment Groups (APG) (DRGs for outpatient services provided at hospital)

Hospital Outpatient Prospective Payment System (HOPPS)—In 2000, HOPPS was implemented to pay for procedures performed at a hospital on an outpatient basis. These mainly included outpatient surgeries, radiology and diagnostic procedures, clinic visits, laboratory visits, and emergency services. The Ambulatory Payment Classification (APC) devises all outpatient pay visits into 300 procedural categories. Each APC is assigned to a relative payment which is weight based and uses the median cost of services within the APC. The APC reimbursement is adjusted for geographical variations in wages and demographics. APC reimbursement is bundled for services such as surgeries that include anesthesia, drugs, supplies, and recovery room charges.

Outpatient Facility Payment Systems

- Straight charges
- Discount percentage of charges
- Percent of Medicare
- Case rates
- Capitation
- Outpatient prospective payment system (OPPS)

Outpatient Prospective Payment System (OPPS)—In 2000, OPPS was implemented to pay for procedures performed on an outpatient facility basis. These mainly included outpatient surgeries, radiology and diagnostic procedures, clinic visits, laboratory visits, and emergency services. The APC and payments are based upon the same philosophy as the HOPPS.

Other Facilities Reimbursement

Medicare Reimbursement to Other Providers—The Balanced Budget Act of 1997 was passed with anticipation to control costs and other healthcare services including skilled nursing facilities (SNF), home health agencies (HHA), and outpatient prospective payment system (OPPS). Three Prospective Payment System (PPS) programs for reimbursement were implemented in 1998 as follows:

Skilled nursing facilities (SNF)—The Balanced Budget Act (BBA) of 1997 modified how facilities are paid for SNF services. SNFs are paid a comprehensive per diem under PPS. The PPS utilizes Resource Utilization Groups (RUG) created by CMS for the determination of payments. RUGs are similar to DRGs or APCs but are solely used for SNFs. There are 66 RUGs that were created and reimbursement specific to each facility and adjusted based on (1) geographical differences in wage rates and (2) patient case mix.

Home health agencies (HHAs)—Under PPS, Medicare pays HHAs a predetermined base payment, and the payment is adjusted for (1) health condition and care needs of the beneficiary, (2) geographical differences in wages, and (3) adjustment for the health condition or clinical characteristics, and service needs of the beneficiary are referred to as the case-mix adjustment. This adjustment for the case-mix adjustment is with home health resource groups (HHRG), which are very similar to RUGs. The home health PPS will provide HHAs with 60-day episode payments for each beneficiary.

Other Terms and Definitions

Chargemaster—Normally found in a hospital and is the overall list of a hospital's charges displaying the hospital billing codes and the related charges.

Case rate—Reimbursement is a payment to the provider based on a predetermined fee that includes all care regardless of any additional costs and resources utilized.

Carve-outs—These are services that are not part of a general negotiated fee schedule with an MCO. A carve-out may be a special drug or an implant that have very high costs. A special agreement is made on that drug or implant outside of the normal agreed-upon fee rates.

Churning—The practice of seeing patient or providing services that are more than necessary or not medically warranted in order to increase revenue.

Cost-shifting—The process of charging some MCOs more than others with the premise to make up for low-paying MCOs such as Medicare and Medicaid.

Exclusion—Services that have no coverage under a MCO contract.

Encounter—An encounter is any time a service takes place such as a visit to a provider or a laboratory test. Each is considered 1 encounter.

Outliers—This is a service that falls out of a range. A hospital contract with an MCO may determine that costs for procedures over a certain cost will be considered outliers and will be paid at a different rate or schedule.

Pay for performance (P4P)—This is a payment system of reimbursement that pays clinicians bonuses based on predetermined performance measures. Incentives are to improve the quality of care, improve outcomes, improve patient safety, and promote cost-effective care.

Risk pool—The "withholds" are placed into an "account" that is called the risk pool. This money is used to pay for services that are utilized over the budgeted amount or paid to the provider if the MCO is under budget.

Withhold—In capitated payment systems, part of the reimbursement is not paid to the provider and is held by the MCO. This amount is referred to as the "withhold amount."

Facility fee—Hospitals that own physicians' offices or ancillary facilities can add a charge called a facility fee.

Further Reading

Barton P. Understanding the U.S. health services system. Chicago, IL: Health Administration Press; 2010.
Buchbinder S, Shanks N. Introduction to health care management. Burlington, MA: Jones & Bartlett Learning; 2012.
Cleverley W, Cleverley J, Song P. Essentials of health care finance. Sudbury, MA: Jones & Bartlett Learning; 2011.
Finkler S, Ward D. Accounting fundamentals for health care management. Sudbury, MA: Jones and Bartlett; 2006.
Kongstvedt P. Managed care. Boston: Jones and Bartlett; 2004.
Marcinko D, Hetico H. The business of medical practice. New York: Springer; 2011.
Huss W, Coleman M. Start your own medical practice. Naperville, IL: Sphinx; 2006.
Niles N. Basics of the U.S. health care system. Sudbury, MA: Jones and Bartlett; 2011.
Reiboldt J. Financial management of the medical practice. Chicago, IL: American Medical Association; 2011.
Shi L, Singh D. Delivering health care in America. Sudbury, MA: Jones & Bartlett Learning; 2012.
Shi L, Singh D. Essentials of the U.S. health care system. Burlington, MA: Jones & Bartlett Learning; 2013.
Solomon R. The physician manager's handbook. Sudbury, MA: Jones and Bartlett; 2008.
Sultz H, Young K. Health care USA. Burlington, MA: Jones & Bartlett Learning; 2014.
Yousem D, Beauchamp N. Radiology business practice. Philadelphia: Saunders/Elsevier; 2008.

Chapter 14
Corporation and Hospital Structures

Abstract This chapter will discuss corporation and hospital business structures. There are many different types of business or corporation structures that can be formed, and each type of structure has a different purpose and ramifications related to ownership, taxes, and liabilities for the owners of the corporation. General business structures can be personally owned, a legal corporation, or a partnership. Hospitals are business corporations and can be structured differently depending on the type of business and structure of their ownership. Hospitals also differ as to whether they are a for-profit status or a not-for-profit status. Each type of business or corporation structure will be reviewed in this chapter, as well as all forms of hospitals that are established at the time of this publication. Some of the advantages and disadvantages will be given of each possible structure. Healthcare administrators should have a general understanding of these different businesses and hospital structures as they can affect every decision made in business in regard to the operations, regulations, income, and expenses of the business.

Corporations

The most common forms of business structures in use in the United States are a sole proprietorship, C corporation, S corporation, general partnership, limited liability company (LLC), and limited partnership. Each one has differentness in complexity, ease of setup, cost, liability protection, periodic reporting requirements, operations, taxation, and advantages and disadvantages. Choosing the right business form requires a delicate balancing of competing characteristics.

R.V. Bucci, *Medicine and Business: A Practitioner's Guide*,
DOI 10.1007/978-3-319-04060-8_14, © Springer International Publishing Switzerland 2014

Sole Proprietorship

A sole proprietorship is an unincorporated company owned and often operated by a single individual or a married couple. This is the simplest and most common business structure to start a business. There is no legal distinction between the business and the person(s) owning it. Corporation papers do not have to be filed for a sole proprietorship, but the name of the business must be registered in the state corporation. This type of business will only be taxed at the level of the owner(s), whereas the business and the owner are considered one. The business will still follow all regulations set by state and federal authorities and obtain the licenses and other requirements required for the type of business.

Advantages

- Easiest and least expensive.
- Owners can mix business and personal assets and report one personal income tax for a year.
- Owners have complete control over their business without having to consult others.

Disadvantages

- The owners are personally liable for all debts, obligations, and liabilities of the business.
- There can be challenges trying to raise capital for the business since the owners are fully liable for the business.
- Many companies, including healthcare insurance companies and managed care companies, will only contract and do business with corporations legally formed.
- May not be a good option for healthcare businesses as the owner's 100 % liability in the company could mean bankruptcy from as little as one malpractice lawsuit.

Corporation or C Corporation

The corporation is an independent legal entity owned and controlled by a group of shareholders and managed by a board of directors or trustees. The shareholders will own stock in the business. The corporation is separated from the shareholders of the business under a "corporate veil" which separates the liabilities of the business from shareholders. Corporations are more complex than other businesses since they have costly administrative fees, legal requirements, and more complex tax obligations. A corporation must be legally formed and registered with the secretary of state of one of the United States. It does not have to be registered in the same state as a corporation is doing business in. A corporation is taxed at both the corporate level and the individual level and called "double taxation." The owners of a corporation can be any individual or any business.

Advantages

- Since the owners of the business and the business itself are separate, the shareholders are not personally liable for the actions of a business and the shareholders personal assets are protected.
- The corporation can raise capital easier by selling more stock in the business.
- The corporation files taxes separate from the owners.
- Corporations can offer more benefits for employees.
- No limit to the number of shareholders.
- Corporations have an unlimited life.
- Corporations can easily transfer ownership through transfer of shares.

Disadvantages

- Corporations are taxed twice, once at the corporation level and once at the individual level.
- The operations of a corporation can be more costly and time-consuming to start and operate.
- Corporations are highly regulated by federal, state, and local governments and require increased paperwork, record keeping, and management.
- Must hold annual meetings and keep a corporate record book.

S Corporation

An S corporation or S corp is a special type of corporation which is created by an IRS tax election. The S corporation is very similar to the C corporation except that the profits and losses of the business are passed from the corporation to the owners and filed as personal taxes. The main purpose of the S corporation is to avoid double taxation of a normal C corporation. To form an S corporation, the business must incorporate in a state and then file an IRS Form 2553 with the federal government. The liabilities of the shareholders are also limited to their investment in the business, and the corporation shields their personal liabilities with the corporate veil.

S corporation eligibility has special requirements. To qualify for S corporation status, the corporation must meet the following requirements:

- Be a domestic corporation
- Has only allowable shareholders:
  - Individuals.
  - Eligible trusts, estates, and tax-exempt corporations, notably 501(c)(3) corporations, are permitted to be shareholders.
  - Not be an ineligible corporation, i.e., certain financial institutions, insurance companies, and domestic international sales corporations.
  - May not include partnerships, corporations, or nonresident alien shareholders.

- Has no more than 100 shareholders
- Has one class of stock

Advantages

- Eliminates the double taxation of corporation with taxation only the personal level
- Separation between personal liability and corporation liability
- Limited liability for shareholders

Disadvantages

- Special rules for shareholders of S corporations
- Must have annual meetings and record meeting minutes
- Certain rules requiring shareholders to receive reasonable compensation for their duties

Partnership

A partnership is a single business entity in which there are two or more partners sharing the ownership. Each partner contributes to the business different aspects including money, property, skills, and expertise. All partners will share in profits and losses of the business. A partnership is relatively easy to set up like a sole proprietorship, and there are usually no state filing requirements. It is highly recommended to have a partnership agreement between the partners to regulate who will make business decisions, how disputes will be decided, how partners and ownership interests can change, and how profits and losses will be divided.

There are three general types of partnerships:

General partnership—This type of partnership assumes that the profits, liabilities, and management duties are equally divided among all partners. If an unequal distribution is to be agreed upon, then this should be documented in the partnership agreement.

Limited partnership—These are also known as limited liability partnerships. They are more complex than general partnerships. A limited partnership is composed of one or more general partners and one or more limited partners. The general partners jointly manage the business and fully share profits and losses. The limited partners are usually not involved in the day-to-day operations of the business, and their liabilities and profits and losses of the business are limited to their percentage of interest in the business. Limited partnerships must be filed legally with the state in which it is operated.

Limited liability partnership (LLP)—This is a partnership where all the partners in the business have limited liabilities. They exhibit the elements of both partnerships and corporations by having the ease of formation and regulations of a partnership and limited liabilities of the corporation. This type of business structure is normally used by professionals such as accountants and attorneys.

Joint Ventures—These businesses behave as a general partnership but are limited to a period of time or a single project. Joint ventures are normally based on a single business transaction. Individuals or companies choose to enter joint ventures to combine strengths, minimize risks, and increase competitive advantages in the market. Joint ventures are initiated by the two or more parties completing a shareholder or operating agreement which specifies their obligations, risks, and goals.

All partnerships need to register their business with articles of incorporation within the state and established a business name. Some partnerships choose to operate under a different name or fictitious name rather than the registered name. This firm will then be doing business as (DBA) their fictitious name.

Partnerships must file an annual information return to report income, deductions, gains, and losses. The partnership itself does not pay taxes but pass on the income and losses to its partners for taxation purposes. The partnership will provide copies with a schedule K-1 (Form 1065) which is a report of the profits and losses of the business for each partner to be used to file taxes on their own personal taxes.

Advantages

- Generally inexpensive and easy to form
- Less formal structure and rules than a corporation
- Generally easier to gain capital since the partners are invested in the success of the business
- Ability to use strengths and resources of all partners
- Do not have a minimum tax amount as required by corporations

Disadvantages

- Partners are subjected to personal liability for their appropriate share of the business.
- Disagreements among partners occur more often, and resolutions may be challenging.
- Partners receive profits and losses that are derived from their equity in the business and not how much effort, time, and resources are extended by the partners. This can make an uneven balance.
- Individual partners must bear the responsibilities of the actions of their other partners.

Limited Liability Company (LLC)

An LLC is a hybrid type of legal business structure that provides the limited liability features of a corporation and the tax and operational advantages of a partnership. Members of the LLC are referred to as members and can be a single individual, two or more individuals, or corporations and other LLCs. LLCs have been increasingly popular in formations due to their limitations of personal liabilities and the ease of business operations. All profits and losses of the business are passed on to their members and are filed about their personal tax returns. There are certain requirements for an LLC:

- The name of the LLC must be different from any existing LLC in the state and is required to have "LLC" or "limited liability company" attached to it.
- Articles of organization must be filed with the secretary of state of the state you are doing business in.
- Some states require an operating agreement that shows the percentage of interest, allocation of profits and losses, and member's rights and responsibilities.

Advantages

- Do not require annual meetings and less record-keeping rules.
- There are fewer restrictions on profit sharing within an LLC, as members distribute profits as they see fit.
- Independent legal structure separated from their owners.
- Separates personal assets from business debts.
- Limited number of members.
- Governed by operating agreements.

Disadvantages

- Limited life of an LLC as when one member leaves, the business may be dissolved.
- Partners are considered self-employed and must pay self-employment taxes.
- Not allowed in certain states for certain professions.
- States require fees in periodic filings.

Hospital Types

Hospitals come in different makes and models based on different categories including ownership, profit status, teaching, size, and other characteristics. Below are some of the variations along with some extended definitions.

Ownership Type

For-profit private
Not-for-profit private
Public

Government Status

Federal government facility
State or local government facility
Nongovernmental facility

Teaching Status

Teaching hospital
Academic healthcare center hospital
Nonteaching hospital

Level of Care

Secondary hospital
Tertiary hospital
Teaching hospital

Hospital Size

0–99 beds
100–199 bed
200–299 beds
300–499 beds
500+ beds

Organizational Structure

Single community hospital
Freestanding hospital
Member of multi-hospital system
Critical access hospital

Specialty Status

General hospital
Children's hospital
Substance abuse treatment hospital
Psychiatric hospital
Rehabilitation hospital

Geographical Location

Rural
Urban

This section will describe the different types of hospitals.

Public Hospitals

A public hospital is one that is owned by the federal, state, or local government. These are the oldest type of hospitals and contribute to approximate 25 % of hospitals in the United States (Shi and Singh 2013). These hospitals are funded by taxes and supported by their government sponsors.

Federal government public hospitals serve special groups such as military personnel, veterans, and Native Americans. The Veterans Administration (VA) is one of the largest groups of public hospitals owned and operated by the federal government. State government public hospitals are normally limited to mental hospitals and other specialty hospitals such as tuberculosis hospitals.

Local governments such as counties and cities operate hospitals that are open to the general public. These community and city hospitals are funded by state and local taxes and normally support the inner-city indigent and disadvantaged populations.

Some of the larger public hospitals can be affiliated with medical schools where they can play a significant role in training of physicians and other healthcare professionals. Medicare, Medicaid, and state and local tax dollars finance most of the hospital services provided at these facilities. These types of hospitals face many financial challenges and over the past few years have been undergoing closures or privatization. These challenges are due to the financial pressures of our healthcare system in the United States.

Not-for-Profit Hospitals

Not-for-profit hospitals are owned and operated by community associations or other nongovernmental organizations. Their primary mission is to benefit the community in which they are located. They are funded by fees paid by patients, third parties, donations, and endowments. The not-for-profit sector of the hospitals contributes to about 50 % of all US hospitals. The inherent name of "not-for-profit" hospitals is contrary to the fact that all hospitals must generate more revenue than expenses and actually make a profit to stay viable and sustainable to support their mission. Any excess of income over expenses in the nonprofit hospital is reinvested into the hospital and community for improvement and growth.

Not-for-profit hospitals are organized under Section 501C3 of the IRS tax code and are exempt from federal estate taxes and generally do not pay local property or other taxes. These hospitals also have access to tax-exempt bonding and have a tax-deductible status for guest contributions. Public hospitals tend to have the highest proportion of unpaid care of any type of hospital. Some attributes of not-for-profit hospitals include (Buchbinder and Shanks 2012):

- Serves public or community interests.
- Assets belong to the community.
- Exempt from taxes.
- Files an IRS 990 annual corporate tax return.
- No person or private corporation makes a profit.
- Exempt from most business fees.
- Can assess tax-exempt bond markets to raise capital.
- May not participate in political campaigns or influence legislation.
- May not offer stock or stock options to staff.
- Must designate amounts of committee benefit including indigent care.
- Operated by board of trustees that serve with community concerns and without personal financial interests.
- Income above expenses issues to improve hospital services in the community.
- Provides a full spread spectrum of care including prevention, treatment, and education to benefit the members of the community.

For-Profit Hospitals

Private for-profit hospitals can also be referred to as proprietary hospitals or investor-owned hospitals which can be owned by individuals, partnerships, or corporations. They are operated for the financial benefit of the owners or shareholders of the entity. For-profit hospitals account for approximately 20 % of hospitals in United States (Shi and Singh 2013). Some attributes of for-profit hospitals include (Buchbinder and Shanks 2012):

- Serves private interest.
- Assets belong to shareholders.
- Pays federal, state, local, and property taxes.
- Files annual for-profit tax return.
- Profits of the company benefit shareholders.
- Must pay business fees.
- Nonexempt from taxable bond yields.
- May contribute to political campaigns and influence legislation.
- Ability to raise capital and offer stock options to employees.
- Have a very limited obligation to provide indigent care.
- Operated by a board of directors who are shareholders or representatives of shareholders in the company.

Hospital Designations and Types

Community Hospitals

These are the most common types of hospitals in the United States. These hospitals are nonfederal and available to general public. The primary mission is to serve the general community with a wide range of medical services. They are not restricted to serving a particular type of individual or group. This type of hospital can be private or publicly owned and can be profit or nonprofit. Over 85 % of the US hospitals are considered community hospitals (Shi and Singh 2012).

General Hospitals

A general hospital provides a mixture of services including general and specialized services. These types of hospitals normally have an emergency department to care for acute medical cases. A general hospital normally provides diagnostic, treatment, and surgical services for a wide variety of medical conditions. Most hospitals in the United States are considered of the general type. The name "general" is used because these hospitals provide a wider range of services and should not imply that these hospitals are any less specialized or inferior to any specialized hospitals.

Specialty Hospitals

Specialty hospitals are hospitals that deal with specific medical needs in one area of medical practice. They can also be considered niche service hospitals. Some historical types of specialty hospitals can include psychiatric hospitals, rehabilitation hospitals, and children's hospitals. Over the past 20 years, newer specialty hospitals include orthopedic hospitals, cardiac hospitals, cancer hospitals, and women's hospitals. Physician-owned specialty hospitals are the newest trend in specialty hospitals but have come under much federal and public scrutiny for their profit motives.

Psychiatric Hospitals

This type of specialty hospital's main purpose is to provide psychiatric inpatient care and to provide diagnostic and treatment services for patients who have psychiatric-related illnesses. These facilities normally provide psychiatric, psychological, and social work services.

Rehabilitation Hospitals

These types of hospitals specialize in therapeutic services to restore maximum motor functioning to the patient after a disability due to illnesses or accidents. Rehabilitation hospitals require intensive rehabilitation services for the treatment of stroke, spinal cord injuries, trauma injuries, brain-damaging injuries, and other injuries or illnesses that are too extensive for a general community hospital setting. These facilities usually provide physical therapy, occupational therapy, and speech therapy.

Children's Hospitals

Children's hospitals are community hospitals which mainly deal with illnesses of children. These children's hospitals provide neonatal intensive care units, pediatric intensive care units, trauma centers, and transplant services. These hospitals also provide a wide range of services including orthopedic surgery, cardiology, pediatric surgery, cancer treatment, and rehabilitation services. Most children's hospitals are nonprofit and located in major metropolitan areas. They are normally associated with medical schools and academic medical colleges.

Osteopathic Hospitals

Osteopathic hospitals focus on a holistic approach to care. Doctors of osteopathic medicine (DOs) practice a whole-person approach, which means they consider both the physical and mental needs of their patients. They emphasize diet and better environmental factors that influence health as well as manipulation of their body. Their focus is in preventive care.

Teaching Hospitals

A teaching hospital is designated as a hospital having one or more graduate residency programs approved by the American Medical Association.

Academic Medical Centers

These are hospitals organized around a medical school. Besides the training of physicians, research and clinical investigations are a large focus of the hospital.

Outpatient and Freestanding Facilities

Throughout the history of healthcare, there has been a gradual movement of healthcare services from inside a hospital to an outpatient- or community-based setting. There were several patient-centered reasons for this trend including convenience for patients to receive services closer to their home or work, consumer preferences for convenient services, increasing ability to care for patients in outlying and less densely populated areas, and increases in technology that allow these outside services to be rendered in this type of setting. Business reasons for transforming from hospital-based services to freestanding centers include increased reimbursements, lower startup costs and lower cost of operations, growth and geographical control for healthcare systems, and entrepreneurial business opportunities. There are various types of outpatient- or freestanding-type facilities across the country. These facilities can be owned and operated by hospital systems, physician groups, or independent entities and can be organized as for profit and not for profit.

Hospital Outpatient Clinics—Many hospitals and healthcare systems have a network of outpatient services available to patients in the community. This trend has developed for growth of a health system and also due to fierce competition in the healthcare industry. Hospitals have moved their operations to more convenient locations to capture a patient base and also gain downstream referrals to the hospital for inpatient, surgical, and other hospital-based procedures and services needed by their patients. These hospital outpatient clinics can provide locations for employed physicians to practice in primary and specialty services, diagnostic imaging and lab services, pharmacies, outpatient surgery centers, wellness centers, and a host of other services. There has been a financial incentive for the growth of hospital-owned outpatient clinics to take advantage of the increased reimbursements from the hospital outpatient prospective payment system (HOPPS) that developed in 2000, which allows hospital systems to add a "facility" charge in addition to the service provided for increased revenue.

Urgent Care Centers—Urgent care centers began opening in the 1970s. The centers provide care for walk-in patients for basic primary care services to minor emergencies. The centers are normally used by patients for emergent or non-routine episodic reasons. They have become popular due to the convenience of walking in without an appointment and receiving services, convenience of locations, and the extended evening and weekend hours. Many of these facilities will also have diagnostic tests available including radiology and laboratory services.

Convenient Care Clinics—These clinics begin to develop in early 2000 and can be described as scaled-down urgent care centers that are located in convenient locations such as grocery stores and drugstores. These clinics are staffed normally by a nurse practitioner, a physician assistant, and less frequently a physician. The idea for these clinics is to see patients who have easy to diagnose acute conditions, examine and diagnose them in 15 min, and then give the patients the opportunity to purchase a prescription or over-the-counter medication near the clinic. The benefits of these companies are:

- No appointment necessary
- Convenient hours and access
- Affordable care
- In and out in 15 min
- Health screenings and prescription services
- Vaccines and flu shots

The top three treatments for these clinics are inner ear infections, strep throat, and urinary tract infections. These clinics also provide a host of other services including immunizations, CLIA waived laboratory procedures, and sports physicals. Pioneers in this type of business were the MinuteClinic, The Little Clinic, and the QuickClinic. Today, the two largest companies that sustained the business are MinuteClinic and Take Care Clinic.

Ambulatory Surgical Centers (ASC)—These are freestanding surgery centers independent of hospitals that can be owned by hospitals, physicians, or independent entities. These normally provide a full range of services that can be performed on an outpatient basis and do not require overnight hospitalization.

Federally Qualified Community Health Centers (FQHC)—These are federally funded and community-based primary healthcare centers that originated in the 1960s. They were established for rural or underserved communities across the country. Their characteristics are as follows:

- Formed under Section 330 of the Public Health Service Act.
- Focused on the needs of the underserved.
- Comprehensive primary care services.
- Federally funded.
- Community involvement.
- Partnership between public and private sectors.
- Specialized programs for migrant workers, the homeless, and residents of public housing. Sliding-fee scale payments are based on income.
- 340B prescription program services—Family practice, internal medicine, obstetrics/gynecology, pediatrics, behavioral health, chiropractic, family dentistry, general surgery, geriatric medicine, neurology, ophthalmology, optometry, oral surgery, orthopedic surgery, otolaryngology, physical medicine and rehabilitation, podiatry, psychiatry, and sports medicine. The center for health and wellbeing includes, but is not limited to, acupuncture, aquatic exercise, exercise physiology, hypnotherapy, massage therapy, nutrition education, pain management, and Reiki therapy.

Home Care—Home care services is healthcare delivered to the patients at their homes as opposed to the patient leaving their home for service. Home health services typically include nursing care, medication monitoring, short-term rehabilitation, homemaker services, transportation and shopping assistants, and providing medical supplies and equipment including oxygen tanks, walkers, etc. Home healthcare services are supported by both public and private health insurance companies.

Hospice Services—These are comprehensive medical services for terminally ill patients with life expectancy of 6 months or less. They address the special needs of dying persons and families. Hospice services include medical, psychological, and social services delivered in a holistic context. Their two areas of emphasis are pain and symptom management and psychosocial and spiritual support.

Outpatient Long-Term Care Services—These are normally services provided within a nursing home. They provide two main types of services. One service is an adult day care center provided by healthcare professionals normally during the normal workday. The second function is case management which can be a wide range of services including physical therapy, occupational therapy, or speech therapy.

Public Health Services—These are healthcare services provided by local health departments. The type and amount of services offered will vary by location and municipality. Normal programs or services included in public health service centers are well-baby care, venereal disease clinics, family planning services, tuberculosis screening and treatment, mental health services, immunizations, and other services of this nature.

Free Clinic—A free clinic is a private, nonprofit, and community-based organization that provides medical care at little or no charge to low-income, uninsured, or underinsured persons. These are staffed volunteer healthcare professionals and partnerships with other health providers. Many also provide a full range of primary care and care for chronic conditions, with some providing pharmacy and dental services.

Other Settings—There are a host of other types of outpatient or freestanding healthcare facilities businesses that are in the healthcare marketplace. The most popular models are diagnostic imaging centers, durable medical equipment sales and services, laboratory centers, cardiac catheterization centers, chemotherapy or radiation therapy centers, physical therapy, occupational therapy, speech therapy, gastrointestinal centers, mental health or behavioral health centers, and pain clinics. These can be independent or owned by a healthcare system and can be for profit or not for profit.

Further Reading

Barton P. Understanding the U.S. health services system. Chicago, IL: Health Administration Press; 2010.
Buchbinder S, Shanks N. Introduction to health care management. Burlington, MA: Jones & Bartlett Learning; 2012.
Dahl O. Think business! Phoenix, MD: Greenbranch; 2007.
Hacker S. The medical entrepreneur. [U.S.?]: Nano 2.0 Business Press; 2010.

Harbin T. The business side of medicine. Minneapolis: Mill City Press Inc.; 2013.

Irs.gov. S Corporations. (Online) http://www.irs.gov/Businesses/Small-Businesses-&-Self-Employed/S-Corporations. Accessed 24 Sept 2013.

Keagy B, Thomas M. Essentials of physician practice management. San Francisco: Jossey-Bass; 2004.

Law.cornell.edu. 26 USC § 1361 – S corporation defined|Title 26 – Internal Revenue Code|U.S. Code|LII/Legal Information Institute. (Online) http://www.law.cornell.edu/uscode/text/26/1361. Accessed 30 Sept 2013.

Marcinko D, Hetico H. The business of medical practice. New York: Springer; 2011.

Niles N. Basics of the U.S. health care system. Sudbury, MA: Jones and Bartlett; 2011.

Sba.gov. Choose Your Business Structure|SBA.gov. (Online) http://www.sba.gov/category/navigation-structure/starting-managing-business/starting-business/choose-your-business-stru. Accessed 24 Sept 2013.

Shi L, Singh D. Delivering health care in America. Sudbury, MA: Jones & Bartlett Learning; 2012.

Shi L, Singh D. Essentials of the U.S. health care system. Burlington, MA: Jones & Bartlett Learning; 2013.

Solomon R. The physician manager's handbook. Sudbury, MA: Jones and Bartlett; 2008.

Sultz H, Young K. Health care USA. Burlington, MA: Jones & Bartlett Learning; 2014.

Yousem D, Beauchamp N. Radiology business practice. Philadelphia: Saunders/Elsevier; 2008.

Chapter 15
Physician Employment and Compensation

Abstract Physicians are the key and primary element in any medical business or practice. The practice of medicine cannot occur without a physician, and physicians need to be compensated for their work. There are numerous ways in which a physician can be compensated, and these methods should be understood by both the physician and the administrator of the healthcare business. A physician can be compensated as an independent contractor or as an employee of a hospital, health system, insurance company, or other types of business. Compensation plans will vary depending on the type of business, the position held by the physician, and the structure of the employer. The monetary value or cash paid to a physician is only one aspect of compensation. There other key factors of compensation including vacation time, continuing education, fringe benefit packages, payments for licenses, journals, and hospital dues, etc. Many physicians have been leaving private practice and becoming employed, and this trend has increased in the last few years. Whether a physician chooses to be an independent contractor or an employee, they should know the similarities and differences, as well as the pros and cons of both opportunities. The physician and the administration should understand the basics of the employment contract or independent contractor agreement in order to both benefit and protect the physician and the employer.

Independent Contractor Versus Employee

The first distinction to be made is whether the physician will be an independent contractor or employee. For the purpose of this chapter, an independent contractor will be considered any position that is not officially employed by a physician group, hospital or healthcare system, insurance company, or other types of institution. This physician will be a solo practitioner, a partner in a medical group, or the owner of some type of medical practice and will not have a status as an employee. The distinction between an employee status and an independent contractor status is related to three factors:

Behavioral control—An independent contractor controls their own behaviors, activities, and rules of employment. An employed physician means that someone else will control when, where, and how they provide services.

Financial control—In financial control mean that an independent contractor is the one who controls the money. If physicians control the income and outflows of the finances of business, then they will be considered independent contractors. If the money is controlled by an organization out of their control, then they would be considered employees.

Type of relationship—How the physician is related to the organization is another key aspect to determine employment versus independent contractor status. Most contracts with any organization will state whether the physician is an independent contractor or employee. The second part of the relationship is considered by who pays for fringe benefits, insurance malpractice, and the time period or permanency of the relationship.

The following are factors that can distinguish employed physicians and independent contractors (Marcinko and Hetico 2011):

Employees

- Works at the sight of an employer.
- Uses equipment and instruments owned by the business.
- Cannot directly delegate or hire employees.
- Hours and methods of work are controlled.
- Expenses are reimbursed.
- No or limited investment by physician.
- Compensation is paid in a set pattern.
- Normally works for only one employer.
- Profits and bonuses are limited.
- No need to directly advertise or market themselves.
- The contract states employee relationship.

Independent Contractor

- Work location is determined by the physician.
- Supplies their own equipment and instruments for work.
- Hires and fires employees.
- Hours and methods of work are not controlled.
- All expenses are paid by the physician.
- Greater investment opportunity of the physician in the business.
- Available to work for any number of businesses.
- No defined limit of compensation.

- Free to advertise for business.
- Contractually stated as an independent contractor.

Compensation Models

Compensation models will vary between the private practice arena and in the hospital business type of employment. The following are some different compensation methods and formulas for both types of arrangements.

Independent Contractor or Private Practice

In private practice, normally the only money that comes into a business is compensation for physician services. Whatever is left of this money after the expenses of the business are paid is the only money that can be distributed to the physician owners of the business. The physician practice must determine the best income distribution plan equitable to all physicians.

Equal Distribution—This is the simplest method of income distribution for an employee practice. The amount of money remaining from the income of the practice less the expenses of the business will be divided equally among the physicians of the practice. If a practice brings in $10 million of cash revenues and pays out cash expenses of $4 million, then the physicians of the practice can split up the remaining $6 million between them. While this is the simplest mathematical method of payment, it does not take into account physician productivity factors.

Productivity Distribution—This method pays the physician based on the amount of work they complete. The more a physician works or "practices," the more they can increase their compensation. Productivity methods will vary based on how they are calculated. The simplest method of compensation bases the compensation on the amount of billable dollars produced by the physician. If a physician produces 60 % of the billable charges for a practice, then they should receive 60 % of the cash profits of the business. An alternative way to look at productivity is to calculate the relative value units (RVUs) earned by a physician and determine their percentage of profits in that manner. RVUs are numbers assigned to specific procedures or CPT codes. RVUs are based on (1) the amount of physician work in regard to expertise, time, and skill required, (2) the physician practice expense to operate the business, and (3) an adjustment to compensate for professional liability insurance. Hypothetically an office visit may equate to 1 RVU, and a surgery may count as 10 RVUs. If it is determined that the amount of RVUs earned by one physician is 60 % of the overall RVUs of the practice, then the physician should again collect 60 % of the profits of the business.

Base Plus Bonus Distribution—This is more of a hybrid model between the equal distribution and productivity distribution methods. The physician will first be paid a base salary for their work. If there are profits in the business after expenses are paid, then a bonus plan model can be activated in the business. The remaining cash in the business can be divided among physicians in a number of ways including the equal distribution method or some method which takes into account physician productivity. This method can be a nice alternative to the previous methods since it gives a physician a base salary and takes into account the amount of work performed.

Revenue and Expense Allocation—This is a more complex model of compensation that takes into account both the revenue and expenses of the business. The income allocation is determined as it is in a productivity distribution method. The expenses are assigned to each physician in a similar manner. The physician is assigned expenses relative to the work that they produce. If a physician produces 60 % of the revenue of the business, then they are allocated 60 % of the expenses of the business. Their compensation would be determined by the balance of their revenue less their expenses. Another way to determine expenses is to charge a physician a set rate for any procedure that they perform. The basic office visit may cost the physician $10 for related expenses of that office visit. In this situation, the cash collected for that office visit less the $10 allocated expense can become the physician's compensation for that office visit.

Ancillary Services—This can be an add-on compensation plan to a physician or practice. Some practices have ancillary services such as physical therapy, radiology, or laboratory services. Additional revenue can be distributed to the physician based on the amount of referrals for the services in their own physician practice.

Other Compensation Issues—Other factors in the physician practice can be taken into consideration in determining compensation for physicians. Some of these considerations can include part-time employment which reduced productivity expectations, on-call compensation, medical chairmanships or directorships, speaking or education assignments, and other non-practice types of productivity.

Hospital or Healthcare System Employment

Compensation from a hospital system or other types of health system employment is much different than a private practice. The amount of money available for expenses and physician salaries is not limited by the amount of money generated by physician services. Hospitals have more revenue available since they provide a wider range of services than just physician practice. Therefore, compensation methods for hospitals are not tied to a certain pool of money, and the hospital can be more creative in how it pays its physicians. There are a number of methods that are used to pay physicians as employees in a hospital or health system setting.

Base Compensation—In its simplest form, a base compensation is the amount of guaranteed compensation to a physician over a certain time period. This amount can be considered guaranteed and considered not "at risk." The guaranteed compensation means that the physician will be paid whether or not their productivity supports such a salary. A salary that is not guaranteed would be considered "at-risk" compensation, and the compensation would be tied to some type of productivity measures such as RVUs, collections, or some other metrics which will be discussed in the next section. More commonly, a physician's compensation has both a base compensation and a productivity portion as well.

Productivity Compensation

Most employed physician's compensation plans have some type of productivity model attached to it. The four common productivity models are the RVU model, percentage of collections model, pay band model, and distribution net income model.

RVU Model—The RVU model is the most popular type of hospital-employed physician's compensation existing in today's market. A base compensation may or may not exist with the RVU model. The physician is paid a base RVU dollar rate for each RVU produced. The physician's compensation is calculated by multiplying the base RVUs rate times the number of RVUs produced. A physician hypothetically may produce 4500 RVUs at the base RVU rate of $31 and be paid a total compensation of $139,500 for the period of time calculated. There are two types of RVU models: a single-tiered model and a multiple-tiered model. A single-tier model uses one base RVU dollar rate for all RVUs produced by the physician. A multiple-tier model has different levels of RVU rates based on the type of work done by the physician. This multiple-tier model is more complicated since the appropriate RVUs must be matched to the appropriate base rates for that RVU to be calculated. A physician may hypothetically have three different RVU rates at $31, $41, and $51 depending on what services they are providing. The appropriate RVUs will be matched to the correct RVU tier and then added together for the final compensation amount.

Percentage of Collections Model—This model is very similar to the individual productivity model used for the independent contractor. The employer will base the physician's compensation by a percentage of the collected cash revenues. A physician may be paid 35 % of collected charges of that physician. If $600,000 is collected for the physician's charges, then a physician salary will be $210,000.

Pay Band Model—This model is based on either RVUs or percentage of collections. It is a rolling 12-month calculation that is adjusted every quarter. Every quarter, the last 12-month worth of productivity is compared to industry benchmarks and then is paid to the physician at predetermined levels per their contract. The physician salary can then change every quarter based on increases or decreases in their productivity. This model can be quite complicated to keep track of and can be challenging for both the physician and the employer.

Net Income Model—This model is very similar to the revenue and expense allocation method previously mentioned. A physician's compensation will be based on their percentage of revenue less the assigned expenses for that physician practice. The hospital will assign expenses for the physician's work based on the hospital/

physician employment contract. This model is not as popular as the RVU model since the physician can be at risk for the assigned expenses of this model.

Other Compensations

Employment arrangements with hospitals or other employers can include other forms of compensation. These additional compensations can be based on the missions and goals of the hospital, other duties for leadership responsibilities of the physician, on-call coverage, and administrative-type compensations. Examples of some nonproductive compensations can be as follows:

- Bonuses for expense control, patient satisfaction results, quality, and adherence to duties
- A daily or hourly rate paid for on-call coverage that exceeds the normal level of expected hours
- Additional compensation for duties of chairman or director of the department
- Additional compensation for administrative functions
- Compensation or reduced productivity time in order to perform research and development

Types of Physician and Employment

Pros and Cons of Private Practice and Employment

There are numerous pros and cons of working in a private practice or being employed by a health system. This can be a tough decision for a physician. The recent trend of the country in the last few years has transferred many physicians from their private practice to the hospital-type employment environment. By 2014, it is estimated that 50 % of the physicians in this country will be working for a hospital or healthcare system as an employee (Gottlieb 2013). There are positives and negatives of both types of employment that the physician must consider. Below are some of the considerations:

Pros and Cons of a Private Physician Practice

Pros

- Autonomy of owning your own business.
- Physicians manage and operate the business.
- Uncomplicated decision process.
- Atmospheric culture may be more relaxed with less rules, policies, and procedures.

- Physicians are shareholders in the corporation.
- Greater ability to earn more money by being more productive.
- Greater ability to increase revenue through ancillary services.

Cons

- Need to handle the administrative aspects of the business.
- Physician leaders may be inexperienced in business skills.
- Physicians will be at risk for incomes and liabilities of the business.
- Income can be inhibited or lessened by expected and unexpected expenses.
- Could be more hours of work.
- Incomes may be lower.

Pros and Cons of Hospital Employment

Pros

- Hospital is at risk for expenses of the business.
- Physicians are assured of their incomes.
- Many physicians receive higher incomes.
- Administrative issues are handled by the hospital support team such as human resources, billing, and daily operations.
- More flexibility and freedom and better work-life balance.
- Steady hours and expectations, normally working fewer hours than in a private practice.
- Hospital management understands the healthcare business.

Cons

- Loss of autonomy of running a business.
- May not have the ability to impact major decisions of the business.
- Possible loss of profit from not getting revenue for ancillary services of the business.
- Compensation may change depending on productivity.
- Performance may be judged by metrics such as quality and patient satisfaction.
- Physicians may not fully understand all the terms of their employment contract.
- May not have the ability to pick their staff, facilities, and other resources.

Hospital Employment Contracts: Features and Tips

A physician entering into practice under an employment arrangement will be employed through an employment agreement. All contracts and agreements should be in writing and not in a verbal or oral form. There is a simple rule for documentation: If it is not written down and documented, then it does not exist. This agreement will occur whether it is an employment agreement with a private practice or with a hospital/health system. The physician's attorney and accountant should always be consulted in contract negotiations to verify that the physician is appropriately represented and fairly treated in the contract. There are certain parts of the contract that the physician should pay close attention to as described:

Parties and start date—The first section of the employment contract will be to designate who the employer and the employee are as well as the start date of the agreement. Both parties should verify that the expected start date is realistic since this contract is a binding legal agreement. Physician's medical licenses and the employer's credentialing processes of physicians can take longer than expected and must be considered when setting the start date.

Duties—This is a section of the contract which is very important and establishes the duties, responsibilities, and expectations of the physician in their employment. The amount and hours of work required of the physician should be detailed in this area. Descriptions of duties should be as specific as possible. Generalities and ambiguities can cause disagreements during the time of employment. This section may also include work expectations based on productivity or relative value units. The physician should verify that the productivity expectations are achievable and measurable.

Exclusivity—A binding employment agreement may include a disposition that the physician works exclusively for the employer and can perform no outside duties. This would be an exclusive employment relationship. A non-exclusive agreement means that the physician can seek other employment or "moonlighting" opportunities at other facilities. Oftentimes, the employer will contract the physician to an exclusive agreement, but the physician may seek other duties or employments with the "permission of the employer." If this is the case, then this should be clearly spelled out in the contract. The contract should clearly state any and all restrictions on outside physician employment.

On-call coverage—There should be a section in the employment agreement that states whether or not the physician will be required for on-call coverage or not. If on-call coverage is an expectation, then it should be designated how much coverage is required under the basis of this contract and whether or not there is compensation related to this call coverage.

Compensation—The contract will specifically state how much one will be paid and when one will be paid. The compensation is normally expressed as a monthly or annual base salary. The section may include a sign-on bonus, incentive bonuses for work done while employed, or other specific compensations for other duties outside of the listed duties in the previous section.

The compensation section can also include some of the following:

- Amount of vacation or paid time off (PTO).
- Amount of PTO to attend continuing education courses and conferences. Many contracts allow continuing medical education in addition to the vacation or PTO.

This section will also detail any reimbursement allowances for continuing medical education including registration fees, lodging and travel, and other travel related expenses.

- Any reimbursement allowances for medical licenses, certifications, and hospital physician staff fees, etc.
- Who will pay and/or how much will be paid for licensure for boards, tests, exams, DEA licenses, medical society memberships, dues, hospital medical staff fees, etc.
- Amounts to be reimbursed for relocation expenses.

Term of contract—Normally a contract is specified for a certain time period such as 1 or 2 years. These types of contracts can automatically renew and are considered "evergreen." An evergreen contract will automatically renew unless it is terminated by either party by a specified number of days before the end of the contract. If the contract is not evergreen, then the physician and the employer must create a new contract upon the termination of the previous one. The type of contract termination or renewal language should be clear and understandable by both parties.

Termination—There will be a section of the contract that explains termination before the scheduled end date. Some of the termination features for this section will be:

Death and disability—The contract may terminate on the death or disability of the physician. Disability needs to be defined as an inability to perform essential functions of the job for a set period of time. There should be clear terms as to when the compensation and termination of the employment agreement occurs in a disability situation. The physician should also consider disability insurance before entering any contract and whether or not this disability insurance will be paid by the employer or the employee.

With or without cause—A contract normally carries both a "with-cause" and a "without-cause" paragraph. With-cause termination means that the employer can terminate the employee with no notice for items that interfere with the physician's ability to perform their duties and other specified items. With-cause reasons can be a suspension or loss of a medical license, loss of hospital privileges, exclusion from the Medicare or Medicaid program, inability to obtain malpractice insurance, or conviction of a crime. There can be other items added to this list that can be used by the employer for with-cause termination, and these should be spelled out in this section. A without-cause termination means that the employer can terminate the employee at any time and for any reason that the employer chooses. This without-cause termination is solely based on the employer's discretion to terminate the employee.

Professional liability insurance—It should be designated in the employment contract whether or not the employer will pay for the employee's professional liability insurance. It will also be stated how much the expected limits for this liability insurance will be, regardless of who is responsible for the payment of these fees. The type of insurance should be designated as "claims made" or "occurrence." Claims made means that the physician is covered under the malpractice insurance only as long as the policy is in effect. After the policy is no longer in effect, the physician is no longer covered for any instances that occurred during that time. After termination of the malpractice contract, the physician is still liable for any claims of incidents that occurred during the time of the enforced contract. "Tail" insurance should be purchased to cover any claims filed after the claims-made coverage ends. This tail insurance will cover the physician practice after the previous malpractice claims-made insurance is terminated. For example, if a physician is sued for an incident that occurred with a previous employer and after the previous employer's malpractice is ended, the tail insurance will be used to cover the liability for that incident. Tail coverage can be costly. There should be a designation of whether or not there will be tail insurance paid as part of this agreement. If the type of insurance coverage is called "occurrence," then it means that the professional liability insurance will cover the physician permanently. In the same situation mentioned, if the insurance was an occurrence type, then the physician would not have to purchase tail insurance because he would be still covered with the original insurance.

Benefits—There should be a separate section to include what benefits are included in the employment agreement including health, disability and life insurance, and retirement plans. All benefits should be listed in this area. The employer may include a section that states they can reserve the right to change the benefits at their discretion.

Restrictions and covenant not to compete—Most contracts may include restrictive covenants and covenants not to compete. A covenant not to compete may specify the physician cannot work for a specified group of competitors or a geographical region for a period of time after the contract is terminated. Other restrictions can include a promise not to disclose employer's proprietary and confidential information such as patient and referring physician lists, non-solicitation of any of the current employers and employees, and non-solicitation of any of the employer's patients after the physician's contract is terminated. These noncompete clauses need to be realistic and reasonable for both sides. The penalties for violation of restrictions or covenant not to compete need to be spelled out in this section as well.

Educational loan forgiveness—Employers may agree to pay off the physician's medical education loans in return for the physician agreeing to stay with the employer for a certain length of time.

Equity ownership—Some employers are professional groups, and the physician may have an opportunity to be a partner or shareholder in the company. This section of the contract should specify the terms and requirements to become a partner or shareholder.

Employment agreements are contractual agreements between an employer and employee. These agreements should be reviewed carefully and changed as needed for both the physician and the employer of the physician. All parts and pieces of employment contracts are negotiable.

Further Reading

Adler E. Employees vs. contractors in medical practice: what's in a name?. Employees vs. contractors in medical practice: what's in a name?. Phys Prac. 2013. http://www.physicianspractice. com/blog/employees-vs-contractors-medical-practice-whats-name. Accessed 27 Sept 2013.

Allegiancemedsource.com. Contract tips. (Online) http://www.allegiancemedsource.com/ Contract%20Tips.htm. Accessed 27 Sept 2013.

Beckershospitalreview.com. Hospital employment vs. private practice: what makes sense for Orthopedic Surgeons? [Online] Available from: http://www.beckershospitalreview.com/ hospital-physician-relationships/hospital-employment-vs-private-practice-what-makes-sense-for-orthopedic-surgeons.html. [Accessed 6 Feb 2014]

Aaos.org. The physician as employee: Pros and cons. (Online) http://www.aaos.org/news/aaos-now/sep09/managing4.asp. Accessed 27 Sept 2013.

Cleverley W, Cleverley J, Song P. Essentials of health care finance. Sudbury, MA: Jones & Bartlett Learning; 2011.

Harbin T. The business side of medicine. Minneapolis: Mill City Press Inc.; 2013.

Hacker S. The medical entrepreneur. [U.S.?]: Nano 2.0 Business Press; 2010.

Huss W, Coleman M. Start your own medical practice. Naperville, IL: Sphinx; 2006.

Kongstvedt P. Managed care. Boston: Jones and Bartlett; 2004.

Keagy B, Thomas M. Essentials of physician practice management. San Francisco: Jossey-Bass; 2004.

KevinMD.com. Pros and cons of private practice vs. hospital owned. (Online) http://www.kevinmd. com/blog/2011/05/pros-cons-private-hospital-owned-practice.html. Accessed 27 Sept 2013.

Kreager M. A guide to understanding and negotiating a physician employment contract … from the employee physician's perspective. [e-book] Kreaerlaw.com.; 2007. http://www.kreagerlaw. com/wp-content/uploads/2013/01/GuidetoUnderstandingandNegotiatingaPhysician.

Marcinko D, Hetico H. The business of medical practice. New York: Springer; 2011.

Online.wsj.com. Scott Gottlieb: The Doctor will not see you now—he's clocked out. (Online) http://online.wsj.com/article/SB10001424127887323628804578346614033833092.html. Accessed 27 Sept 2013.

Orthopedic Surgeons?. (Online) http://www.beckershospitalreview.com/hospital-physician-relationships/hospital-employment-vs-private-practice-what-makes-sense-for-orthopedic-surgeons.html. Accessed 27 Sept 2013.

Physicianspractice.com. Hospital employment vs. private practice: pros and cons|physicians practice. (Online) http://www.physicianspractice.com/blog/hospital-employment-vs-private-practice-pros-and-cons. Accessed 27 Sept 2013.

Solomon R. The physician manager's handbook. Sudbury, MA: Jones and Bartlett; 2008.

Reiboldt J. Financial management of the medical practice. Chicago, IL: American Medical Association; 2011.

Yousem D, Beauchamp N. Radiology business practice. Philadelphia: Saunders/Elsevier; 2008.

Chapter 16
Medical Business Law and Regulations

Abstract Healthcare organizations, healthcare administrators, and practitioners need to be cognizant of federal and state regulations and laws that apply to the healthcare business. Violations of some of these laws can result in criminal penalties, civil fines, exclusion from federal and state healthcare programs, loss of hospital privileges, or loss of a medical license from the state medical board. Some of the more significant fraud and abuse laws are the False Claims Act (FCA), the Anti-Kickback Statute (AKS), the Physician Self-Referral Law (Stark law), and the Civil Monetary Penalties Law (CMPL). Federal government agencies including the Office of the Inspector General, Department of Justice, Department of Health and Human Services, and Centers for Medicaid and Medicare Services have enforced these laws to healthcare organizations in every state. An understanding of these laws will help protect healthcare providers from fines, costly defenses, and possible prison time.

False Claims Act (FCA)

The FCA (31 United States Code [U.S.C.] Sections 3729–3733) law created in 1863 protects the government from being overcharged or charged improperly for its services. The law states that it is illegal to submit medical claims to federal healthcare programs such as Medicare or Medicaid that are known or should be known to be false or fraudulent. Under the FCA, no specific intent to defraud the government is required. "Knowing" is defined by the FCA to include both actual knowledge about instances of fraudulent activity and instances where a person acts with deliberate ignorance or reckless disregard for the truth or falsity of information (OIG 2013). Some areas of highest risk for FCA violations to healthcare entities are as follows:

- Services billed and never delivered.
- Bills for nonexistent patients.

- Anti-kickback violations for solicitation or receipt of money, property, or other remuneration for a referral of patients or healthcare services.
- Upcoding of medical claims where the provider bills for more than what was actually done.
- Unbundling of services that should normally be billed as a bundle or package.
- Performing medically unnecessary exams.
- Inappropriate physician investments or compensation arrangements.
- Falsified or inaccurate hospital cost reports to gain higher reimbursements.
- Redlining is a reimbursement scheme where hospitals and/or insurance companies increase their profits by only enrolling the healthiest people.

The FCA also contains a whistle-blower provision that allows private individuals to report suspected false claims acts to the US government. If the government investigates and prosecutes the suspected healthcare provider, then the whistle-blower is entitled to receive a percentage of the monetary recoveries. Common whistle-blowers are current or ex-business partners, hospital or office staff, patients, or competitors. Falsified claims filed with Medicare or Medicaid can result in fines up to three times the amount of the falsified claim plus $11,000 per claim filed. Criminal charges can also be applied including prison time and criminal fines.

Anti-Kickback Statute (AKS)

The Anti-Kickback Statute (42 U.S.C. Section 1320a–7b(b)) is a criminal law created by the Social Security Amendments in 1972 to protect patients and federal healthcare programs from fraud and abuse. Congress, in 1977, enacted the Medicare-Medicaid Anti-Fraud and Abuse Amendments which increased the penalties for fraud and abuse from a misdemeanor level to a felony level while adding a list of penalties. In 1987, the Medicare and Medicaid Patient and Program Protection Act allowed the Office of the Inspector General (OIG) to be given authority to levy civil, as well as criminal penalties for fraud and abuse cases. The statute prohibits the "knowing or willful" acts of individuals or companies from seeking, receiving, or offering remuneration in exchange for referring patients to receive items or services paid by the government programs including Medicare and Medicaid (OIG 2013). Some of these items or services include prescription drugs, supplies, healthcare services, and ancillary services that are payable by federal health programs. Remuneration can include items of value such as cash, travel expenses, meals, excessive compensation for duties or positions, and other items of "value" that can be used to generate referrals to provider. It was not uncommon for providers to be taken to professional sports events and skiing trips or allowed to use a condominium in a resort area in exchange for referrals. This law covers both the providers of the kickbacks and the receivers of the kickbacks as being liable under the AKS. Criminal and administrative penalties for violating the AKS include fines, imprisonment, and exclusion from participation in federal healthcare programs.

Individuals can face fines of $50,000 per kickback, plus three times the amount of the remuneration.

Physicians are likely targets for kickbacks since they recommend what services the patient is to receive, which specialist they can be referred to, what drugs the patient uses, and other referral-type activities. Kickbacks in the healthcare business can lead to increased costs, corrupt medical decision-making, patient steering, and unfair competition advantages. While kickbacks are normally cash- or gift-type inducement, waiving co-payments and deductibles can also be seen as a kickback. Many drug manufacturers and healthcare companies have implemented extensive compliance programs to protect themselves from suspected kickback activities. Nowadays, companies like drug manufacturers don't even give away logo pens to physicians, as opposed to the past when meals, little gifts for physicians and staff, and golf outings were common giveaway items.

Antitrust Acts

The following antitrust laws were implemented to protect the citizens of the United States from the negative effects from monopolies:

The Sherman Antitrust Act of 1890 (15 U.S.C.A. §§ 1 et seq.)—This is the first and most significant of the US antitrust laws. This act prohibits conspiracies or agreements that could possibly restrain trade or business. These include but are not limited to price-fixing, boycotting, bid-rigging and market-allocation agreements, territory allocation agreements among competitors, or using coercive efforts to intentionally harm or injure another party. This act applies to all businesses in the country including healthcare.

Clayton Act of 1914 (15 U.S.C.A. §§ 12 et seq.)—This act prohibits mergers or acquisitions that can weaken competition in the market. This act is applicable to any business in the country and can result in civil penalties.

Robinson-Patman Act of 1936 (15 U.S.C.A. §§ 13a, 13b, 21a)—This act makes it illegal to discriminate in price between two purchasers of products or services of similar quality and grade. This can occur when an organization sells the same product to two different healthcare providers at different prices, and this purchase price can affect competition. The buyer can also be held liable for accepting goods at different prices in order to gain an advantage over its competitors. There is a Nonprofit Institutions Act that provides exceptions to the Robinson-Patman Act allowing hospitals to purchase supplies "for its own use" at discounted prices.

Federal Trade Commission Act of 1914 (15 U.S.C.A. §§ 41 et seq.)—This act prohibits unfair methods of competition. Activities include collusion, price-fixing, large businesses using their size to gain lower prices, and the use of discount differentiation among different sized firms.

Penalties can be very high for antitrust violations in the healthcare business. Violators can have prison sentences of up to 10 years and fines up toward $1 million per person or $100 million for an organization. For civil liabilities, the other party can receive up to three times the damages plus attorney fees. The courts also have the authority to seize any property of unlawful conduct, dissolve unlawful arrangements or entities, or disqualify an unlawfully acquired entity.

Physician Self-Referral Law or Stark Law

The Physician Self-Referral Law (Stark law) (42 U.S.C. Section 1395nn) prohibits physicians and immediate family members of the physician to have ownership or investment interest in a "designated health service" and receive compensation or dividends from that business. The simplest example is if a physician owns or partially owns an imaging center, refers patients to the imaging center for tests, bills a federal healthcare payer such as Medicare or Medicaid for exams, and then receives investor-related payments from the business. A common business in which physicians became investors to earn extra income for their referrals was an MRI center in which the physicians referred business for the MRIs and received payments for being an investor in the business. Designated health services that are illegal include the following (OIG 2013):

- Clinical lab services
- Physical therapy, occupational therapy, and speech language pathology therapy
- Radiology and other imaging services
- Radiation therapy services and supplies
- DME and supplies
- Parenteral and enteral nutrients, equipment, and supplies
- Prosthetics, orthotics, and prosthetic devices and supplies
- Home health services
- Outpatient prescription drugs
- Inpatient and outpatient hospital services

The Stark law is a liability statute which means that no proof of "intent to violate" the law is required. Simply referring to a designated health service in which there is ownership violates this law. Penalties for violation of the Stark law include fines and exclusion from federal health programs.

There are exceptions to the Stark law's provisions. There are approximately 35 exceptions that are acceptable financial relationships and allow a physician to refer to an entity for the provision of designated health services. The two categories affected by these exceptions normally deal with ownership/investment interest and compensation arrangements. There are common requirements that apply to Stark law exceptions:

- The arrangement must be signed by all parties specifying the services, space, and equipment covered in the deal.

- The compensation for the arrangement must be set in advance and be consistent with fair market value.
- The compensation cannot be determined by the volume or value of the referrals.
- The arrangement must be commercially reasonable.
- The business must serve a legitimate business purpose.
  The most commonly used business exceptions of the Stark laws are:
- Ownership in publicly traded securities and mutual funds
- In-office ancillary services
- Rentals of office space and equipment
- Personal service arrangements
- Bona fide employment agreements
- Payments by physicians
- Certain arrangements with hospitals
- Physician recruitment

While this list is limited by terms of exceptions, these are the most common used exceptions by healthcare providers. There are specifications for each of these exceptions which should be reviewed in depth by the healthcare provider if they are interested in pursuing. An attorney should always be consulted when starting a new business to protect you and your company from entering into an illegal business activity.

Criminal Health Care Fraud Statute

The Criminal Health Care Fraud Statute (18 U.S.C. Section 1347) prohibits knowingly and willingly attempting to and/or executing a scheme to:

- Defraud any healthcare program.
- Obtain any money or property owned by or under the control of any healthcare benefit program.

Penalties for violation of the Criminal Health Care Fraud Statute can include fines, imprisonment, or both.

Special Fraud Alerts

The OIG is constantly gathering information about fraud and abuse practices in the healthcare industry. Special fraud alerts are areas where activity has increased or heightened in a certain area of fraud and abuse. These special fraud alerts are the OIG's way to notify the industry that certain abusive practices have come into light, and the OIG plans to pursue, prosecute, and bring forth administrative action as appropriate for these violations. These alerts also can be used as a tool by healthcare providers to examine their practices and verify that they are not in any violation of fraud and abuse. There have been 12 special fraud alerts since 1994:

- Joint venture relationships
- Waivers of co-payments or deductibles under Medicare part B
- Hospitals in certifying referring physicians
- Prescription drug marketing schemes
- Arrangements for provision of clinical laboratory services
- Home healthcare fraud
- Fraud and abuse in nursing home facilities in the provision of medical services
- Fraud and abuse in nursing home arrangements with hospices
- Fraud and abuse in the provision of services in nursing facilities
- Physician liability and certification of medical equipment and supplies and home health services
- Rental of office space in physician offices
- Telemarketing by durable medical equipment suppliers

Emergency Medical Treatment and Active Labor Act (EMTALA)

This is also known as the antidumping act. It prevents emergency rooms from refusing treatment or transferring patients to another facility because of the patient's inability to pay for treatment. This act mandates that an appropriate medical screening exam is given to any patient presenting to an established provider of emergent or urgent care. If the exam shows an emergency condition exists, the patient must be either treated or admitted as inpatient. The act also restricts emergency room personnel from discussing financial returns information about the patient until after the medical exam has been performed and the emergent condition has been stabilized. Centers for Medicaid and Medicare Services have the authority to enforce EMTALA and impose financial penalties to providers who do not obey the act. The Office of the Inspector General also has authority to impose sanctions against violators. Violators can incur money penalties up to $50,000 per violation and also have their Medicare program participation terminated.

Exclusive Statute

The Office of the Inspector General (OIG) is legally required to exclude individuals and entities from all federal health programs who were convicted of the following crimes and offenses (OIG 2013):

- Medicare or Medicaid fraud and abuse.
- Patient abuse or neglect.

- Felony convictions for other healthcare-related fraud, theft, or financial misconduct.
- Federal convictions for unlawful manufacture, distribution, prescription, or disposing of controlled substances.
- The following are some additional offenses which the OIG can use at its discretion to decide whether exclusion is deemed necessary:

  - Misdemeanors related to health fraud
  - Other Medicare or Medicaid misdemeanors for fraud convictions
  - Suspension, revocation, or surrender of a license to provide healthcare services based on professional competence, professional performance, or financial integrity
  - Provision of substandard or unnecessary services
  - Submissions of false or fraudulent claims to a federal healthcare program
  - Engaging in unlawful kickback arrangements
  - Defaulting on health education loans or scholarship obligations

Exclusion by the OIG from participation in federal healthcare programs includes Medicare, Medicaid, as well as other programs such as TRICARE, the Veterans Health Administration, and the Indian Health Services. Anyone excluded by the OIG cannot directly bill for treating Medicare and Medicaid patients or bill indirectly as a facility or group for an excluded employee or independent contractor providing services for that facility or group. It is a responsibility of the billing entity or employer to ensure that your organization is not billing for a physician that is excluded by the OIG. This responsibility requires screening of all current and prospective employees or contractors for your organization. There is an online "Exclusion List" of excluded individuals and entities at the OIG's exclusion website.

Government Enforcement Programs

Office of the Inspector General (OIG)—This protects the integrity of the HHS' programs including Medicare and Medicaid for the health benefit of its beneficiaries. The OIG performs these duties through a national network of audits, investigations, inspections, and other related functions. The inspector general has the authority to exclude individuals and organizations who have engaged in fraudulent or abusive activities from this patient in a federal healthcare program. The OIG maintains a list of excluded parties called the list of excluded individuals/entities that can be located at https://oig.hhs.gov/exclusions on the Internet.

Civil Money Penalties Law (CMPL)—This authorizes the Secretary of Health and Human Services to impose civil money penalties and program exclusions for fraud and abuse involving the Medicare and Medicaid programs. The fraud and abuse cases that can be enforced are:

- Filing claims with a federal healthcare program for an item or service that was not provided as claimed or is false or fraudulent

- Violating the Anti-Kickback Statue by offering or paying remuneration to induce the referral of a federal healthcare program service or soliciting or receiving remuneration in return for the referral of federal healthcare program services
- Filing claims for services for which payment may not be made under the Stark law

Penalties can range from $2,000 to $100,000 for each occurrence. The inspector general needs only to prove liability by a "preponderance of the evidence" rather than the more demanding "beyond a reasonable doubt" standard. The healthcare provider can be held liable for its own negligence and the negligence of its employees. Intent to defraud the federal healthcare agencies is not required for prosecution.

Health Care Fraud Prevention and Enforcement Action Team (HEAT)—HEAT is a combination partnership between the Department of Justice (DOJ) and the Department Health and Human Services (DHHS) to build on and strengthen its existing programs to combat Medicare and Medicaid fraud by investing in new technologies and resources to further prevent fraud and abuse. HEAT has created the Stop Medicare Fraud website, which provides information on how to identify and protect against Medicare fraud. This is located at http://www.stopmedicarefraud. gov on the Internet.

Health Insurance Portability and Accountability Act (HIPAA) Program—This is also known as the Kennedy-Kassebaum Act, and its purpose is to provide expanded powers and increased funding to the federal government in areas of healthcare fraud and abuse in both the public and private sectors. Their purpose is to search out and prosecute suspected fraud and abuse cases. This regulation has three purposes: (1) to protect and enhance the rights of consumers by providing them access to their health information and controlling the use of that information, (2) to improve healthcare quality in the United States and to restore trust in the US healthcare system and its providers, and (3) to improve the efficiency and effectiveness of our healthcare delivery system by creating a national program to protect health privacy in the United States.

Healthcare Fraud and Abuse Control (HCFC) Program—This program is a joint effort between the Office of the Inspector General and the Department of Justice. The purpose is to coordinate federal, state, and local enforcement to control healthcare fraud and conduct investigations regarding the delivery and payment of healthcare services, monitor Medicaid and Medicare exclusions, anti-kickback law, and civil money penalties.

Medicare and Medicaid Integrity Programs—These are two independent programs authorized by the Department of Health and Human Services to contract with nongovernmental organizations to carry out the mission of fraud and abuse detection, cost reports audits, utilization review, provider payment determinations, and provider education. Their mission is to (CMS 2013):

- Hire contractors to review Medicare and Medicaid provider activities, audit claims, identify overpayments, and educate providers and others on Medicare and Medicaid program integrity issues.

- Provide effective support and assistance to states in their efforts to combat Medicare and Medicaid provider fraud and abuse.

Health Care Fraud and Abuse Control Account (Section 1817 of the Social Security Act/42 U.S.C. 1395i(k))

This is a special "bank" account or fund established by the Department of Health and Human Services and the Department of Justice to fund activities related to administration in the operation of healthcare fraud and abuse control programs. While this program will be funded mostly by federal appropriations, a certain portion of funds collected from healthcare fraud and abuse penalties and fines will also be used to fund the account.

Beneficiary Incentive Program

This program encourages beneficiaries to report any suspicious billing activities in healthcare that has been personally observed. Medicare beneficiaries are encouraged to call, report, and possibly be rewarded for occurrences that result in action. If at least $100 is collected as the result of the report, a portion of the amount collected may be paid to the individual who reported the information. Another part of the program encourages individuals to submit suggestions to the Department of Health and Human Services to improve the efficiency of the Medicare program. If a suggestion is adopted and results in a savings of a Medicare program, the individual submitting the suggestion will receive a portion of the savings.

National Practitioner Data Bank (NPDB)

This program was originally established by Title IV of the Health Care Quality Improvement Act of 1986, Public Law 99-660. The purpose of this data bank is to improve the quality of healthcare in the United States with the help from the state licensing boards, professional societies, hospitals, and other healthcare entities. The program will collect and store data in regard to malpractice history and adverse actions including licensure, clinical privileges, professional society membership actions, drug enforcement agency actions, and exclusions from federal healthcare programs. This program is intended to improve healthcare quality, protect the public, and reduce healthcare fraud and abuse.

Compliance Programs

As one can see from the information in this chapter, there are many opportunities for fraud and abuse in the healthcare sector. Providers of healthcare services including physicians, hospitals, and other providers need to be cognizant of possible fraud and abuse situations and guard themselves against conducting business in a noncompliant manner. The OIG has been encouraging healthcare organizations to participate in a voluntary compliance program since 1998. The OIG has developed and published voluntary compliance program guidance focused on several areas of the healthcare industry. The OIG's belief is that an internally based compliance program by the healthcare provider can be effective in monitoring and adhering to applicable laws, regulations, and program requirements. The OIG has published program guides that can be found on the OIG website at http://www.hhs.gov/oig. All compliance programs recommended by the OIG have seven components which are as follows (oig.hhs 2013):

- Conducting internal monitoring and auditing
- Implementing compliance and practice standards
- Designating a compliance officer or contact
- Conducting appropriate training and education
- Responding appropriately to detected offenses and developing corrective action
- Developing open lines of communication
- Enforcing disciplinary standards through well-publicized guidelines

Further Reading

Ama-assn.org. Federal fraud abuse laws. (Online) http://www.ama-assn.org//ama/pub/physician-resources/legal-topics/regulatory-compliance-topics/health-care-fraud-abuse/federal-fraud-enforcement-physician-compliance/federal-fraud-abuse-laws.page. Accessed 4 Oct 2013.

Cms.gov. Medicaid Integrity program – general information – centers for medicare and medicaid services. (Online) http://www.cms.gov/Medicare-Medicaid-Coordination/Fraud-Prevention/MedicaidIntegrityProgram/index.html?redirect=/medicaidintegrityprogram/. Accessed 4 Oct 2013.

Dahl O. Think business! Phoenix, MD: Greenbranch; 2007.

Harbin T. The business side of medicine. Minneapolis: Mill City Press Inc.; 2013.

Hacker S. The medical entrepreneur. [U.S.?]: Nano 2.0 Business Press; 2010.

Oig.hhs.gov. Compliance Guidance|Compliance|Office of Inspector General|U.S. Department of Health and Human Services. (Online) https://oig.hhs.gov/compliance/compliance-guidance/index.asp. Accessed 2 Oct 2013.

Oig.hhs.gov. Fraud & Abuse Laws|Physician Roadmap|Compliance|Office of Inspector General|U.S. Department of Health and Human Services. (Online) http://oig.hhs.gov/compliance/physician-education/01laws.asp. Accessed 30 Sept 2013.

Pozgar G. Legal aspects of health care administration. Sudbury, MA: Jones & Bartlett Learning; 2012.

Teitelbaum J, Wilensky S. Essentials of health policy and law. Sudbury, MA: Jones and Bartlett; 2007.

Chapter 17
New Government Initiatives

Abstract There has been a great deal of activity in the area of federal healthcare policies over the last few years. These changes have and will affect how healthcare services are accessed, managed, and paid for. Health records and protection of individual health records have also seen legislation passed. Also, further changes to patient record keeping and billing, coding of medical records, and the electronic storage of these records are occurring. This chapter will discuss some of the newer activities in healthcare policy that have made changes in healthcare industry over the last few years, making alterations currently and more changes in the future. These changes will affect every part of healthcare; and the administrators and physicians need to be aware of these legislative actions. Some of the healthcare policy changes include the Patient Protection and Affordable Care Act, accountable care organizations, the Health Insurance Portability and Accountability Act, the Health Information Technology for Economic and Clinical Health Act, and the change of diagnosis codes from ICD-9 to ICD-10. While some of these new laws have already been implemented and in effect, there are many actions from these laws to be enacted over the next few years. These laws have impinged and will impinge on all participants in healthcare system including the insured, the uninsured, providers of healthcare services, payers of healthcare services, taxpayers, businesses, and all US citizens.

Patient Protection and Affordable Care Act

The Patient Protection and Affordable Care Act (PPACA or ACA) was signed into law by President Barack Obama on March 23, 2010. The ACA has also been called "ObamaCare" by many in the country. The intent of this law was to expand healthcare coverage to all Americans, reduce the costs of healthcare, increase patient protection, and eliminate or control many of the challenges in their current healthcare system. The ACA went in effect in 2010, and the implementation schedule ranges from 2010 until after 2014 with the majority of the changes occurring during by January 1, 2014. The government will take a much larger role in control and operations of the US healthcare system. In 2014, all US citizens will have access to affordable insurance options according to the current schedule of the ACA. The ACA will affect all parts of the healthcare system including the beneficiary, providers, and payers, and each of these parties will be affected differently. Some of the effects on the stakeholders of the ACA are as follows.

The Insured

Insured citizens of our country will see many changes with this new law. There will be added benefits to beneficiary's insurance coverage, preexisting illnesses clauses will be removed, there will be more opportunities to utilize health spending accounts and flexible spending accounts, and citizens will see more opportunities to make insurance carrier changes with greater ease and a number of other initiatives. On the counter side, there will be more situations for employer-paid insurance to be discontinued due to rising costs to the employer, the Medicare beneficiary will see fewer benefits, and our healthcare system will be stressed due to inadequate healthcare professionals to care for all the new citizens with healthcare insurance. This increase with new Medicaid and new "healthcare exchange" insurance beneficiaries could overwhelm the current healthcare system with the millions of new citizens with insurance benefits which may lead to decreases in the amount and the quality of care received today.

The Uninsured

There are approximately 50 million citizens in our country that are uninsured as of 2010 (Tate 2012). Of these 50 million people, 37 million are American citizens that will be able to receive healthcare insurance with the ACA of some form, and 13 million are illegal aliens that will still be unable to receive healthcare benefits in this country. All of these 37 million people, 14 million will qualify to enroll in Medicaid, 14 million can enroll in a subsidized insurance plan in the new healthcare exchange program, and 9 million can purchase an unsubsidized plan through the healthcare exchange.

Senior Citizens

All seniors on the Medicare advantage plan will see benefit cuts in this program in the next decade. The projected cuts of these benefits will be $455 billion (Tate 2012). On the plus side for seniors, the Medicare prescription drug program will increase its benefits and will reduce the "doughnut hole" effect on Medicare citizens.

Taxpayers

Taxpayers under the ACA will see increases in new taxes directly and indirectly imposed to cover the funding of the new regulations. There is also a capital gains tax on citizens that earn more than $250,000 for a married couple. There will be some increased taxes on capital gains of home sales above $500,000. These new taxes involve every American in the United States in some manner.

High-Wage Earners

Any Americans who earn more than $200,000 per year will see Medicare tax deduction increase from the current 1.4 % level to 2.35 % (Tate 2012). Also, any Medicare beneficiaries with a high income will see increases to their premiums for Medicare part D.

Small Businesses

Businesses with 25 or fewer employees will benefit from this ACA law as they will have access to healthcare insurance plans through the healthcare exchanges starting in 2014. This will allow small businesses and their employees to gain insurance coverage at reduced rates.

Physicians

The ACA law has much potential to decrease income to physicians in both the private independent contractor model and the healthcare system employment model. The increase in the citizens with health insurance will also exemplify the shortage of primary care physicians while increasing the physician's workload with new Medicaid and healthcare exchange patients. The increase in new beneficiaries is expected to be over 30 million beneficiaries by the final implementation of this ACA (Tate 2012). The country may also see a continued trend of physicians leaving the private practice and becoming employees in hospital and healthcare systems. Other physicians will join accountable care organizations (ACOs) in order to be part of the system.

Healthcare Professionals

With the increase in new enrollees with healthcare insurance, the healthcare professionals such as a nurse should have more job stability and possibly a higher salary since there may not be enough healthcare professionals to care for all new citizens with insurance. On the negative side, the increase in new insurance beneficiaries could exaggerate shortages of healthcare professionals and decrease the quality and amount of care provided to.

ACA Changes by Year

The ACA has a scheduled implementation which starts in March of 2010 and continues for a number of years. Most of the changes were expected to occur between March 2010 and January 1, 2014, but part of the implementation schedule has been altered with some extensions into 2015 and beyond. More of these extensions are likely to occur. The following is a summary of legislative actions of the ACA:

2010

- Preexisting conditions for children—The new law prevents all children 18 years of age and under from being denied for health insurance due to preexisting health conditions.
- Child healthcare extension—All healthcare insurance companies must now offer family coverage to allow defendant to children to stay on the parent's policy until the age of 26 years old.
- Annual and lifetime spending limits—Insurance companies are prohibited from imposing lifetime dollar limits on most benefits such as hospital stays, emergency care, auditory patient services, and prescription drugs.
- Preventive and emergency services—Health insurers and healthcare plans, which are not grandfathered in, are required to provide certain preventive healthcare services. These services are to be provided without any deductibles, co-payments, or coinsurance. These services include immunizations recommended by the Advisory Committee On Immunization Practices of the Centers for Disease Control and Prevention, preventive care and screening for infants and children, adolescents supported by guidelines from the Health Resources and Services Administration, preventive care screenings for women supported by the Health Services and Services Administration, and recommendations from the US Preventive Services Task Force. Also the health insurance companies must cover emergency medical conditions without preauthorization, co-payments, deductibles, or coinsurance.
- Prohibition under rescissions of healthcare insurance—The insurance provider is not allowed to rescind any individuals' healthcare insurance unless that individual is involved in some type of insurance fraud or misrepresentation.
- Internal and external appeals process—All insurance providers are required to meet minimum standards in regard to internal review processes for an appeal of an adverse benefit decision and also implement an external review process that would be consistent with the consumer protection in the National Association of Insurance Commissioners.

- Preexisting condition insurance plan—The ACA established a temporary high-risk pool for individuals that are unable to find health insurance or credible coverage for any insurance company. This pool will exist until January 1, 2014. After this, other parts of the ACA will be able to cover these individuals.

2011

- Prescription drug discounts—Seniors reaching the current "doughnut hole" region will receive a 50 % discount on buying Medicare part D-covered brand-name prescription drugs to decrease this challenge of purchasing prescription drugs.
- Free preventive care for seniors—Certain free preventive services and wellness visits for seniors will be established.
- Insurance premium reductions—85 % of all premium dollars collected by insurance companies must be spent on healthcare services for their beneficiaries. Any amounts under 85 % of the premiums not spent on healthcare services for beneficiaries must be returned to the insured in the form of a rebate.
- Integrated health systems—There is a host of new opportunities and new incentives for hospitals and physicians to join together and integrate their services.
- Over-the-counter drug payments—Health spending accounts and flexible spending accounts can no longer be used to pay for over-the-counter drugs.
- Restaurant nutritional information—Any restaurants with more than 20 locations are required to provide nutritional information in calorie amounts under menus.

2012

- Formation of accountable care organizations (ACOs) that will improve and coordinate patient care for all citizens. This will be discussed in the next section.

2013

- Increase payments to primary care physicians—Primary care physicians will receive Medicaid payments of not less than 100 % of the Medicare payment rates in 2013.

2014

- Increase Medicaid access—All Americans who earn less than 133 % of the poverty level ($14,000 for an individual and $29,000 for a family of four) will be eligible to enroll Medicaid. States will receive 100 % federal funding for the first 3 years to support this expanded coverage, phasing to 90 % federal funding in subsequent years. This is effective on January 1, 2014 (ASPA 2013).
- Healthcare exchanges—A healthcare insurance marketplace will be established in 2014 at either the state or federal level for healthcare coverage. These healthcare exchanges will lower the cost of insurance to individuals, increase consumer's choice, standardize insurance plans, increase consumer protection, and take advantage of economies of scale's limited number of insurance companies. Consumers will be able to receive federal subsidies for their health insurance

for individuals who earn between 100 and 400 % of the federal poverty level (400 % of federal poverty level is approximately $43,000 for the individual or $88,000 for the family of four). Individuals can review options and sign up for healthcare coverage starting on October 1, 2013, to be effective on January 1, 2014. Citizens access the government website for the healthcare exchanges which is www.healthcare.gov or call the Health Insurance Marketplace at 800-318-2596.

- Employer-mandated insurance coverage—All employers who employ more than 50 employees are required to provide these employees some type of healthcare coverage by January 1, 2014, or they will be subject to tax penalties. The type and amount of the insurance are not mandated at this point in time. The tax credit issued to his employers will be 50 % of the cost of healthcare paid by the employer. The fines for employers not supplying health insurance to their employees will be approximately $2,000 per worker (Tate 2012).
- This requirement was delayed in June of 2013 to have a new effective date of January 1, 2015. Further studies and requirements for this part of the ACA will be reviewed and republished.
- Individual insurance responsibility mandate—All citizens of the United States will be required to maintain some type of qualified insurance coverage or pay a penalty, unless exempted. This is effective January 1, 2014, and the maximum penalties are $285 in 2014, $975 in 2015, and $2,085 in 2016 for noncompliance (Tate 2012).

Funding of the ACA changes is driven from Medicare payment cuts to providers, increased taxes to hospitals in drug companies, noncompliance ACA penalties, taxes on high-cost insurance plans, and some other revenue sources such as education cuts and community-assisted living reductions. The ACA is a very complicated and controversial issue in this country. Changes are occurring every day to the original ACA and modifications are made. Changes are occurring at the time of the printing of this book and more are expected in the future.

Accountable Care Organizations (ACOs)

Section 3022 of the Affordable Care Act added Section 1899 to the Social Security Act which establishes Medicare Shared Savings Programs (CMS 2013). The Centers for Medicaid and Medicare Services (CMS) finalized rules on October 20, 2011 to coordinate doctors, hospitals, and other healthcare providers to provide coordinated care for Medicare patients (CMS 2013). The *Accountable Care Organization* (ACO) is the first Shared Savings Program introduced. ACOs are special integrated groups of providers to take responsibility for the overall healthcare of a defined group of Medicare population. This Medicare Shared Savings Program certifies providers to lower healthcare costs and increase standards of quality of care for the beneficiaries. This program encourages hospitals, physicians, and other healthcare providers to create new entities together as an ACO and be held responsible for the health and care for individuals, reduce the growth rate of healthcare spending, and improve the health of Medicare beneficiaries.

The idea for an ACO is to take total responsibility for a large group of Medicare beneficiaries in the matter what their healthcare needs are from immunizations to catastrophic illnesses. The minimum size group of Medicare beneficiaries will be 5,000 enrollees. Some of the roles of organizational structures possible for ACOs are as follows. (ACO professionals being defined as hospitals, physicians, and other healthcare providers)

- Partnerships and joint ventures between hospitals and ACO professionals
- Hospitals employing ACO professionals
- ACO professional in group practice arrangements
- Networks of individual practices of ACO professionals
- Other Medicare providers and suppliers as determined by the secretary

Some specific business structures and rules for the participation of business structures for the ACOs are as follows (CMS 2013):

- The ACO forms must be a separate legal entity from any other entity of the ACO participants.
- The ACO must operate in the state in which it is organized.
- Complete a Medicare ACO application describing how the ACO plans to deliver high-quality care and lower expenditures for the Medicare beneficiaries.
- The ACO must be formed for the purpose of receiving and distributing shared savings, risk sharing, and bonus sharing opportunities with the CMS. The ACO will be responsible for establishing, reporting, and complying with quality health criteria and quality performance standards.
- Accept responsibility for a minimum of 5,000 Medicare fee-for-service beneficiaries for participation in the ACO.
- Notify included ACO beneficiaries of their enrollment in the program.
- Accept the metrics and methodologies for savings as set by the CMS for risk sharing.
- Accept final rule quality performance measures and methodologies set by the CMS for linking quality and financial performance with the concept of delivering coordinated and patient-centered care.
- The governing board of the ACO must include 75 % memberships of the ACO participants, include one Medicare beneficiary who does not have a conflict of interest, and operate a similar manner of a nonprofit health plan.

The overall goal of an ACO is to deliver high-quality seamless healthcare for Medicare beneficiaries rather than fragmented care seen in the normal fee-for-service healthcare system. If the ACO meets the program's quality performance standards, then it will be eligible to receive a bonus or share of the savings assigned to that Medicare beneficiary group. If it is unable to meet these expectations, then the ACO will share the loss and repay Medicare a portion of the losses.

At the time of this publication, it was estimated that there were more than 400 ACOs in the United States located in 49 out of 50 states (Muhlestein 2013). Delaware is the exception and has no ACOs. The largest majority of ACOs are found in the states of California, Florida, and Texas. There are more ACOs forming and evolving in our country today. ACOs are still a work-in-progress and the amount of success or failure they will have is undetermined and at this time.

Health Insurance Portability and Accountability Act (HIPAA)

The Health Insurance Portability and Accountability Act (HIPAA) of 1996 was created to improve the efficiency and effectiveness of the healthcare system in the United States. This law provides federal protections for individuals in regard to identifiable health information held by healthcare organizations and their business associates and gives patients rights in regard to that information. This law also permits the disclosure of this health information when needed for patient care and other healthcare purposes. The US Department of Health and Human Services published the final ruling for HIPAA in 2000 but it was later modified in 2003. The rule sets national standards for protecting the confidentiality, the integrity, and the availability of electronic protected health information (hhs.gov 2013). This act took effect on April 14, 2003, and healthcare providers were required by law to adopt policies and procedures to give patients "rights" in regard to their confidential information. This statute overruled any preexisting state or federal laws concerning the confidentiality of medical records. These patient's "rights" included:

- The right of consent to use or disclose the patient's demographic information including the patient's name, address, social security number, and any other information that could be used to identify an individual.
- The right of a description of the intended uses and disclosures of this demographic information.
- The right to authorize or withhold authorization for uses and disclosure purposes other than for treatment and billing of the medical visit. An example would be to use a patient's information for fundraising of medical facility.
- The right to receive a statement listing all disclosures of patient's demographic information specifically to who, when, what, and why disclosures were made.
- The right to require restrictions on the uses and disclosure of patient information.
- The rights to have all these restrictions apply in verbal, written, and electronic form.
- These rules must be written in a language and form that can be easily understood by all patients and families.

In 2009, the American Recovery and Reinvestment Act made changes to the original HIPAA privacy security rules implemented in 2003. These new rules expand the obligations of healthcare providers to protect patient's protected health information (PHI), increase obligations to other individuals and companies known as "business associates" that have access to PHI, and increase penalties for violations of any of these obligations. The new rule became effective on March 23, 2013, and healthcare businesses had until September 23, 2013, to be in compliance of these new rules. Some of the highlights of the new rules to be in effect are (AMA 2013):

1. Breach notification requirements—The obligation to notify patients if there is a breach of their PHI is expanded and clarified under the new rules. Breaches are now presumed reportable unless, after completing a risk analysis and applying HIPAA four factors, it is determined that there is a "low probability of PHI compromise." The four factors are:

   • The nature and extent of the PHI involved including the possibility of re-identification
   • Who the unauthorized person was in which the information was disclosed or used by
   • Whether or not the PHI was actually disclosed or reviewed
   • The extent to which the risk of protected information was mitigated

2. The original HIPAA maybe set forth standards for all healthcare facilities to post Notice of Privacy Practices (NPP). The NPP informs patients of their privacy rights with respect to their personal health information, and this information must be available to every patient entering that healthcare business. Healthcare practices must now update their NPP to reflect the changes set forth above, including those related to breach notification, disclosures to health plans, and marketing and sale of PHI. To the extent that healthcare providers are engaged in fundraising, the providers will also have to amend their NPP to inform patients of their participation in these activities. The patient has their right to opt out of those communications. As the rules state, these are all material changes and healthcare providers will have to post the revised NPP and make copies available at their office to all new patients. Physicians who maintain a website should update the NPP on their website as well. The new rules also eliminate requirements to include information on communications concerning appointment reminders, treatment alternatives, or health-related benefits or services in NPPs, but the rules do not require that that information is removed either.

3. The new rule expand the definition of individuals and companies who must be treated as business associates to include: patient safety organizations and others involved in patient safety activities, health information organizations such as e-prescribing gateways, and personal health record vendors. Thus, physicians must review their relationships and determine if they must enter new business associate agreements (BAAs) with these entities or others that create, receive, store, maintain, or transmit PHI on their behalf.

Health Information Technology for Economic and Clinical Health (HITECH) Act

The American Recovery and Reinvestment Act of 2009 was enacted as part of its Charter, the Health Information Technology for Economic and Clinical Health (HITECH) Act, on February 17, 2009. The purpose of this act was to promote the adoption and meaningful use of health information technology, specifically electronic health records (EHR). EHR is defined as a systematic collection of electronic health information about individual patients or populations. The HITECH provisions are specifically designed to provide necessary assistance and technical support to healthcare providers, enable the coordination and alignment within and among states, establish connections to the public healthcare communities for emergencies, and guarantee that the workforce is properly trained and equipped in order to be made meaningful to users of the EHR. As part of the HITECH Act, the following programs are to be created and supported by this act (Sultz and Young 2014):

- Beacon Community Program to assist communities in building their health information technology infrastructures
- Consumer eHealth Program to assist Americans to access their own personal health information and use a tool to participate in their own healthcare
- State Health Information Exchange Cooperative Agreement Program to assist states in establishing the exchange of health information among healthcare providers in hospital systems in their regions
- Health Information Technology Exchange Program to establish regional centers of education and training for healthcare providers to use electronic health information technology
- Strategic Health IT Advanced Research Projects to fund research projects to overcome challenges of EHR implementations

Included in the HITECH Act was $20.8 billion to be used in an incentive program called "meaningful use" for eligible professionals including physicians and hospitals (hhs.gov 2013). There is a Medicare and Medicaid Incentive Program in which hospitals and physicians must adopt, implement, upgrade, and demonstrate meaningful use of certified EHR with the end goal to improve patient care. Eligible professionals are able to receive up to $44,000 in the Medicare EHR incentive program and up to $63,750 in the Medicaid EHR incentive program. The Medicare program is a 5-year program operated and funded by the federal government, and the Medicaid program is a 6-year program funded by the federal government but administered by individual states. To receive full benefits from this program, the eligible providers must apply and begin certification by 2012. After this point, the benefits will be reduced each year.

To receive the EHR incentive benefits, the providers must demonstrate that they are using information "meaningfully" as guided by the standards and objectives of the Medicaid and Medicare EHR incentive programs. If a provider fails to implement the EHR in their practice by January 1, 2015 and not demonstrate meaningful use, then Medicare will impose payment penalties in the form of federal healthcare program fee schedule reductions.

ICD-10

The International Classification of Diseases (ICD) is the international standard diagnostic classification for all general medical purposes. ICD codes are used to apply a numeric or alphabetic code to a medical condition or procedure. ICD-9 codes have been around for approximately 30 years and are used in the process of applying diagnosis codes to a patient's medical conditions and procedures. A sample code for pneumonia will look like 782.3 for the ICD-9 code. ICD-9 codes are 3–5 alphanumeric characters. There are approximately 18,000 ICD-9 codes that are in existence in the United States.

In 2008, the Department of Health and Human Services proposed new code sets to be used for reporting diagnoses and procedures and to be implemented on October 1, 2013. The implementation of this change in ICD codes was delayed 1 year until October 1, 2014. The ICD-10 codes would be the new codes and replace the ICD-9 system. The ICD-10 codes are significantly different. There are two types of ICD-10 codes: ICD-10-CM and ICD-10-PCS. ICD-10-CM is the diagnosis classification for use in all US healthcare treatment settings. These codes are 3–7 alphanumeric characters, and there are approximately 60,000 of these codes. The ICD-10-PCS is a procedure classification system to be used in all inpatient hospital setting periods. These codes are seven alphanumeric characters and there are approximately 72,000 of these codes.

The ICD-10 codes are designed to be more specific than the ICD-9 codes. These new codes will detail laterality such as left and right body parts, the exact location of the condition, whether the activity was an initial or subsequent encounter, and whether the episodes were chronic or acute. The ICD-9 system may have only used one diagnosis code for a visit to a doctor, whereas the new ICD-10 system may use 10 codes for the same visit. These codes will have a major impact on medical practices in order to implement the coding of encounters, bill the encounters, and train physicians, allied health professionals, and support staff to properly use the ICD-10 system. An example of the new system is explained by Bucci (2011):

> Dr. Jones sends his patient John to the radiology department for an X-ray of his nasal bones. John's pet turtle bit him and, distracted by the pain, John walked into the lamppost in the driveway of his mobile home, causing him to break his nose and develop a headache.
>
> In the coming world of ICD-10, we'll actually have—perhaps unbelievably—several ICD-10 codes in play for a case such as this one: W59.21XA, Bitten by turtle, initial encounter; W22.02, Walked into lamppost; Y92.024, Driveway of mobile home as the place of occurrence of the external cause; S02.2, Fracture of nasal bones; and G44.311, Acute posttraumatic headache intractable.

As one can grasp from this example, the new system will be quite complicated and will require many resources and education to be used properly. Failure to properly code patients in the future will cause delayed reimbursements and possibly lost revenue. In addition to these challenges, there are some benefits for the US healthcare system. According to CMS (2011), the purposes of the change to ICD-10 are measuring the quality, safety, and efficacy of care; designing payment systems and processing claims for reimbursement; conducting research, epidemiological studies, and clinical trials; setting health policy; operational, strategic planning and designing of healthcare delivery systems; monitoring resource utilization; improving clinical, financial, and administrative performance; preventing and detecting healthcare fraud and abuse; and tracking public health and risk. In order to prepare and change current systems in the medical practice, the provider can follow these steps (Bucci 2011):

- Become familiar with the CMS website for ICD-10 (www.cms.gov/ICD10).
- Perform a SWOT (strengths, weaknesses, opportunities, threats) analysis in your department on the basis of the current state of employees, IT, and environment.
- Determine your department's future statement (what you intend to achieve) for ICD-10 implementation.
- Form a strategic business plan detailing the strategy to move to the future statement.
- Gain buy-in from management.
- Implement your strategy.
- Test, measure for successes and failures, and always improve.

There will be costs associated with the changes, as well as reimbursement challenges after October 1, 2014. The cost for this change will be fully assumed by each provider, which includes training, IT and billing program changes, and hiring of additional personnel. The changes will also have financial effects after the ICD-10 change occurs. Providers are expected to see rejected claims and delays in claims processing and reimbursements. The provider must prepare for a reduced cash flow after the transition takes place.

Further Reading

AMA. The Health Insurance Portability and Accountability Act (HIPAA) Omnibus Final Rule Summary. American medical Association. (Online) http://www.ama-assn.org/resources/doc/washington/hipaa-omnibus-final-rule-summary.pdf. Accessed 20 Sept 2013.

ASPA. Key Features of the Affordable Care Act By Year|HHS.gov/healthcare. (Online) http://www.hhs.gov/healthcare/facts/timeline/timeline-text.html. Accessed 19 Sept 2013.

Barton P. Understanding the U.S. health services system. Chicago, IL: Health Administration Press; 2010.

Buchbinder S, Shanks N. Introduction to health care management. Burlington, MA: Jones & Bartlett Learning; 2012.

Cms.gov. EHR Incentive Programs – Centers for Medicare & Medicaid Services. (Online) http://www.cms.gov/Regulations-and-Guidance/Legislation/EHRIncentivePrograms/index.html?redirect=/EHRIncentivePrograms/. Accessed 20 Sept 2013.

Cms.gov. Accountable Care Organizations (ACO) – Centers for Medicare & Medicaid Services. (Online) http://www.cms.gov/Medicare/Medicare-Fee-for-Service-Payment/ACO/index.html?redirect=/aco/. Accessed 19 Sept 2013.

Cms. (2013). Untitled. (Online) http://www.cms.gov/Medicare/Medicare-Fee-for-Service-Payment/sharedsavingsprogram/Downloads/ACO_Summary_Factsheet_ICN907404.pdf. Accessed 20 Sept 2013.

Fox News. White House releases proposed new rules for ObamaCare employer mandate after delay. (Online) http://www.foxnews.com/politics/2013/09/05/white-house-releases-proposed-new-rules-for-obamacare-employer-mandate-after/. Accessed 19 Sept 2013.

Health Affairs Blog (2013). Continued growth of public and private accountable care organizations. (Online) http://healthaffairs.org/blog/2013/02/19/continued-growth-of-public-and-private-accountable-care-organizations/. Accessed 20 Sept 2013.

Hhs.gov. HIPAA Administrative Simplification Statute and Rules. (Online) http://www.hhs.gov/ocr/privacy/hipaa/administrative/index.html. Accessed 20 Sept 2013.

Hhs.gov. HITECH Act Enforcement Interim Final Rule. (Online) http://www.hhs.gov/ocr/privacy/hipaa/administrative/enforcementrule/hitechenforcementifr.html Accessed 20 Sept 2013.

Hhs.gov. HITECH Act Enforcement Interim Final Rule. (Online) http://www.hhs.gov/ocr/privacy/hipaa/administrative/enforcementrule/hitechenforcementifr.html. Accessed 20 Sept 2013.

Niles N. Basics of the U.S. health care system. Sudbury, MA: Jones and Bartlett; 2011.

Kongstvedt P. Essentials of managed health care. Burlington, MA: Jones and Bartlett Learning; 2013.

Muhlestein D. Health affairs blog. Continued growth of public and private accountable care organizations. (Online) http://healthaffairs.org/blog/2013/02/19/continued-growth-of-public-and-private-accountable-care-organizations/. Accessed 20 Sept 2013.

Nytimes.com. Log In – The New York Times. (Online) http://www.nytimes.com/2013/07/03/us/politics/obama-administration-to-delay-health-law-requirement-until-2015.html?pagewanted=all&_r=0. Accessed 19 Sept 2013.

Radiologytoday.net. ICD-10 and its impact on radiology. (Online) http://www.radiologytoday.net/archive/rt1211p10.shtml. Accessed 20 Sept 2013.

Healthit.gov. HITECH Act – the Health Information Technology Act|Policy Researchers & Implementers|HealthIT.gov. (Online) http://www.healthit.gov/policy-researchers-implementers/hitech-act-0. Accessed 19 Sept 2013.

Shi L, Singh D. Delivering health care in America. Sudbury, MA: Jones & Bartlett Learning; 2012.

Shi L, Singh D. Essentials of the U.S. health care system. Burlington, MA: Jones & Bartlett Learning; 2013.

Sultz H, Young K. Health care USA. Burlington, MA: Jones & Bartlett Learning; 2014.

Tate N. Obamacare survival guide. West Palm Beach, FL: Humanix; 2012.

Index

Printed by Publishers' Graphics LLC
ASO140415.15.18.6